Prescribing in Dia

Prescribing in Diabetes

Jill Hill and **Molly Courtenay**

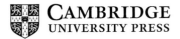

CAMBRIDGE
UNIVERSITY PRESS

CAMBRIDGE UNIVERSITY PRESS
Cambridge, New York, Melbourne, Madrid, Cape Town,
Singapore, São Paulo, Delhi

Cambridge University Press
The Edinburgh Building, Cambridge CB2 8RU, UK

Published in the United States of America by Cambridge
University Press, New York

www.cambridge.org
Information on this title: www.cambridge.org/9780521713351

First published 2008

Printed in the United Kingdom at the University Press, Cambridge

A catalogue record for this publication is available from the British Library

Library of Congress Cataloguing in Publication data
Hill, Jill.
Prescribing in diabetes / Jill Hill and Molly Courtenay.
   p. ; cm.
Includes bibliographical references and index.
ISBN 978-0-521-71335-1 (pbk.)
1. Diabetes – Chemotherapy. 2. Drugs – Prescribing.
I. Courtenay, Molly. II. Title.
[DNLM: 1. Diabetes Mellitus – drug therapy. WK 815 H646p 2008]
RC661.A1H55 2008
616.4′62061–dc22   2007050176

ISBN 978-0-521-71335-1 paperback

CONTENTS

PREFACE

The introduction of non-medical prescribing has meant that nurses, pharmacists and the professions allied to health are frequently faced with prescribing decisions. This text has been written for healthcare professionals involved in the management of treatment for patients with diabetes. Easily accessible information upon which to base prescribing decisions ensuring safe and effective practice is provided in the form of a single, easy to use, practice-based text.

Chapter 1 describes the various methods available to healthcare professionals for the safe delivery of medicines to patients. The pharmacology underpinning prescribing decisions is explored in Chapter 2. Chapters 3, 4 and 5 explore normal blood glucose regulation and diabetes, supporting lifestyle changes and patient empowerment, and the management of glycaemia by oral hypoglycaemic agents. The remainder of the book addresses insulin therapy (Ch. 6), the management of increased cardiovascular risk (Ch. 7) and acute and long-term complications (Ch. 8). This book, in conjunction with the *Nurse Prescribers' Formulary, British National Formulary, Drug Tariff* and manufacturers' product information sheets, provides an essential guide for those healthcare professionals prescribing in the area of diabetes.

ACKNOWLEDGEMENTS

The authors thank the following people for reviewing this book:

Roytun Bibi and Shanaz Mughal (*diabetes specialist nurses*),

Dr Waqar Malik (*community consultant diabetologist*),

Louise Mitchell (*diabetes specialist podiatrist*),

Theresa Smythe (*diabetes nurse consultant*),

Heena Jabbar (*smoking cessation adviser*),

We would also like to thank J. Hemsey for the photography.

The Diabetes Prescriber Network supported by Jill Hill and Molly Courtenay has been set up at Reading University. The Network aims to:

- support the continuing professional development of healthcare professionals who prescribe in the area of diabetes
- provide a forum for peer support and exchange of ideas and information
- share good practice

The Network holds 3 meetings a year (free to members) and provides members with a quarterly printed newsletter.

The registration fee to join the network is £20. For further information about the Diabetes Prescriber Network and to register contact prescribernet@reading.ac.uk

Chapter 1

Methods available for the delivery of medicines to patients

A number of different methods are available to healthcare professionals for the delivery of medicines to patients. These methods include patient specific directions (PSDs), patient group directions (PGDs), independent prescribing and supplementary prescribing. This chapter describes each of these different methods of delivery.

Patient group directions

Legislative changes

Prior to 2000, group protocols were used by nurses and other groups of healthcare professionals to administer or supply medicines to patients. However, the legal basis for these protocols was uncertain and changes in legislation were required to legalise their use. These changes took place in 2000, and group protocols became known as PGDs. The PGDs apply only for use in the National Health Service (NHS), including those services funded by the NHS but provided by the private, voluntary or charitable sectors. They also apply for use by independent hospitals, agencies and clinics registered under the Care Standards Act 2000, the prison health care services, police services, and the defence medical services.

Prescription Only Medicines, Pharmacy or General Sales List items

A PGD, signed by a doctor and agreed by a pharmacist, acts as a direction to a healthcare professional (i.e. midwife, nurse, pharmacist, optometrist, podiatrist/ chiropodist, radiographer, orthoptist, physiotherapist and ambulance paramedics) to supply and/or administer a Prescription Only Medicine (POM) to a patient (using their own assessment of a patients need), without necessarily referring back to a doctor for an individual Prescription. Although General Sales List (GSL) items and Pharmacy medicines can be supplied/administered under a PGD, there is no legal requirement to do so. However, they are used by many Trusts as best practice.

Controlled drugs, antimicrobials, and 'black triangle' drugs

A PGD can be used to supply and administer a wide range of POMs. However, legislative and 'good practice' restrictions are in place with regards to controlled drugs (CDs), antimicrobials and 'black triangle' drugs (i.e. those recently licensed and subject to special reporting arrangements for adverse reactions). With regards to CDs, legislative changes took place in autumn 2003 enabling some of these medicines to be supplied and administered under a PGD. These drugs include Schedule 4 and Schedule 5 controlled drugs (but not anabolic steroids) and diamorphine for cardiac pain by nurses working in accident and emergency and coronary care units in hospitals. Proposals are currently being considered to expand the range of CDs that can be supplied by nurses and pharmacists, and also to change the location and circumstances in which they can supply or administer these medicines (MHRA, 2007).

Antimicrobials can be included within a PGD but consideration must be given to the risk of increased resistance within the general community. A local microbiologist should be involved when seeking to draw up a PGD for these medicines, and approval should also be sought from the Drug and Therapeutics Committee (DTC) or equivalent.

Black triangle drugs and medicines used outside the terms of the Summary of Product Characteristics (SPC), sometimes called 'off label use', may be included in PGDs. However, their use should be exceptional and justified by current best clinical practice. Where the medicine is for children, it is important that specific attention should be given to restrictions on age, size and maturity of the child. Each PGD should clearly state why the product is being used outside the terms of the SPC and the documentation should include the reasons why such use is necessary.

Unlicensed medicines

If a medicine is unlicensed, it should only be administered to a patient using a PSD as opposed to a PGD. However, a medication that is licensed but used outside its licensed indications may be administered under a PGD if its use is exceptional, justified by best practice and the status of the product is clearly described. In addition, sufficient information to administer the drug safely and acceptable evidence for the use of that product should be available.

Dose adjustment under a patient group direction

The dose adjustment of medicines under a PGD is acceptable. However, in order to meet legislative criteria, the dose or maximum dose must be specified: that is, it is necessary for the PGD to specify a single dose or a range up to a specific maximum dose. The pharmacist and doctor that are responsible for signing the PGD must be satisfied that the dose range specified is clinically appropriate. It is also necessary to specify the clinical criteria for selecting a dose within that range. The healthcare professional using the PGD must be competent to make the decision on dose.

Patient specific directions

In a situation where it is not possible to legally use a PGD, for example a supermarket that dispenses medicines, then a PSD can be used to administer a medicine. In this situation, each medicine would need to be prescribed for patients on an individual basis by a registered prescriber on a named patient basis.

Independent and supplementary prescribing

Recommendations by the Department of Health and Social Services were first made in 1986 for nurses to take on the role of prescribing (DHSS, 1986). Eight years later (although limited to district nurses (DNs) and health visitors (HVs)), nurses in eight demonstration sites throughout England began independent prescribing. There are now over 30 000 DNs and HVs qualified to prescribe from a list of appliances, dressings, Pharmacy items, GSL items and 13 POMs included in the *Nurse Prescribers' Formulary* (NPF) for community practitioners.

The introduction of independent extended prescribing in 2002 by the Department of Health (DoH, 2002), and supplementary prescribing in 2003 (DoH, 2003), has further expanded the prescribing powers of both nurses and other non-medical health professionals. Any appropriately qualified registered nurse or pharmacist is able to prescribe any licensed medicine (including off label medicines and some CDs; Box 1.1) independently (provided it is within their area of competence). Proposals to expand the range of CDs that can be prescribed independently by nurses and pharmacists are currently being considered (Home Office, 2007). Additionally, appropriately qualified nurses, pharmacists, allied health professionals (AHPs) and optometrists are able to prescribe any medicine (including unlicensed medicines and CDs) as supplementary prescribers. In contrast to independent prescribing, supplementary prescribing takes place following an initial

---

Box 1.1 Controlled drugs included in the *Nurse Prescribers' Formulary*

- Diazepam, lorazepam, midazolam (Schedule 4 drugs) for use in palliative care
- Codeine phosphate, dihydrocodeine and co-phenotrope (diphenoxylate hydrochloride and atropine sulphate) (Schedule 5 drugs)
- Diamorphine, morphine or oxycodone for use in palliative care
- Buprenorphine or fentanyl for transdermal use in palliative care
- Diamorphine or morphine for pain relief in respect of suspected myocardial infarction or for relief of acute or severe pain after trauma including in either case post operative pain relief
- Chlordiazepoxide hydrochloride or diazepam for treatment of initial or acute withdrawal symptoms caused by withdrawal of alcohol from persons habituated to it.

---

assessment and diagnosis of a patient's condition by a doctor. A clinical management plan (CMP) is then drawn up for the patient. This plan, agreed by the patient and supplementary prescriber (and doctor), includes a list of medicines (within the supplementary prescriber's area of competence) from which the supplementary prescriber is able to prescribe. Supplementary prescribing is best suited to patients with chronic or long-term healthcare needs.

REFERENCES

DoH (2002) *Extending Independent Nurse Prescribing within the NHS in England: A Guide for Implementation.* London: Department of Health.

DoH (2003) *Supplementary Prescribing for Nurses and Pharmacists within the NHS in England.* London: Department of Health.

DHSS (1986). *Neighbourhood Nursing: A Focus for Care (Cumberlege Report).* London: HMSO.

Home Office (2007). *Public Consultation: Independent Prescribing or Controlled Drugs by Nurse and Pharmacist Independent Prescribers.* London: Home Office.

MHRA (2007). *Patient Group Directions* (MLX 336). London: Medicines and Healthcare Products Regulatory Agency.

Nurse Prescribers' Formulary. London: BMJ Publishing and RPS Publishing.

USEFUL RESOURCES

http://www.portal.nelm.nhs.uk/PGD/default.aspx
http://medicines.mhra.gov.uk
http://www.dh.gov.uk

Chapter 2

Pharmacology and decision-making in prescribing

The expansion of prescribing by non-medical healthcare professionals is likely to benefit people with long-term conditions such as diabetes, ensuring that care is both effective and convenient. Given the increasing rates of diabetes, managing it and its complications will be an important part of the workload for many new prescribers.

All prescribers need a good knowledge and understanding of pharmacology and how it influences decisions about the choice of drug; the route of administration, dose and frequency; and the management of potential contraindications, side-effects and interactions with other drugs. Pharmacological treatment of diabetes aims to regulate blood glucose levels using insulin, insulin-stimulating drugs or insulin-enhancing drugs.

This chapter examines the fundamentals of **pharmacokinetics** – how drugs move within the body and are affected by it – and **pharmacodynamics** – the effects drugs have on the body and what moderates these effects. It highlights issues to consider when assessing clients before prescribing medication, using examples from the treatment of diabetes and its complications.

Routes of administration

Drugs can act either locally, mainly after topical administration, or systemically, mainly after oral or parenteral (see below) administration. If a drug acts locally, its effects are confined to a specific area; systemically acting drugs enter the vascular and lymphatic systems for delivery to body tissues. It is possible, however, for topical drugs to have systemic effects, especially if doses are large, frequent or administered over a long period. The administration route affects the **bioavailability** – the proportion of the administered dose that reaches the circulation in effective form. Prescribers need to select the route that will be most clinically and cost effective.

Topical administration

Topical preparations may be applied to the skin, mouth, nose, oropharynx, cornea, ear, urethra, vagina or rectum. They can be administered in a variety of forms: creams, ointments, gels, lotions, aerosols, foams, plasters, powders, patches, suppositories and sprays. In prescribing for diabetes and its complications, the following are commonly used: capsaicin (Axain) cream for peripheral neuropathy pain, alprostadil intraurethrally (MUSE) for erectile dysfunction and ketoconazole (Nizoral) cream for toenail fungal infections.

Oral administration

Oral drug administration (by mouth) is the most common method as it is usually convenient, simple and safe. Solid preparations can be in the form of tablets, capsules, powders, granules and lozenges; liquid forms include solutions, emulsions, suspensions, syrups, elixirs and tinctures. Prescribers managing clients with diabetes and its common complications are likely to be using the following: oral hypoglycaemic agents such as gliclazide, antihypertensive drugs, statins and aspirin.

Parenteral administration

Parenteral administration of a drug refers to its injection or infusion intradermally, subcutaneously, intramuscularly, intravenously, intrathecally and intra-articularly, but not gastrointestinally. It is, therefore, a common method of delivering medication for diabetes. Insulin, as it is a protein, is digested if given orally. It is, therefore, usually given by subcutaneous injection. Sterile preparations for parenteral administration are in the form of ampoules, vials, cartridges or large-volume containers; insulin is most commonly dispensed as disposable pen devices or cartridges to fit reusable pen devices.

Pharmacokinetics: absorption, distribution, metabolism and excretion

After administration, drugs undergo four processes: absorption, distribution, metabolism and excretion. Where and how effectively these processes happen will be influenced by the composition of the drug concerned, its dosage, the client's condition and other therapeutic and environmental issues. The prescriber must consider all of these.

Drug absorption

Drug absorption delivers the drug from the administration site into the circulatory or lymphatic system. Apart from drugs administered intravenously and some topical preparations, nearly all drugs must be absorbed before they can have an effect on the body. All prescribers need to understand how the process of absorption works and what factors affect it in order to select the optimal formulation and route of administration. Intravenously administered drugs are said to be 100% bioavailable as they are administered directly into the circulation. **Bioavailability** is reduced when drugs are administered by other routes as some of the drug molecules are lost during absorption, distribution and metabolism.

Drugs administered orally are absorbed from the gastrointestinal tract, carried via the hepatic portal vein to the liver and undergo some metabolic processes in the liver before they start to take effect; this is known as the **first pass effect**. Some drugs, when swallowed and absorbed, will be almost totally inactivated by the first pass effect, for example glyceryl trinitrate. The first pass effect can, however, be avoided if the drug is given by another route. For example, glyceryl trinitrate can be administered sublingually or transdermally, thus avoiding first pass metabolism by the liver and enabling a therapeutic effect.

For drugs not administered intravenously, several lipid cell membrane barriers must be crossed before the drug reaches the circulation. Lipid-soluble drugs will pass through these membranes more easily than water-soluble drugs. Four major transport mechanisms facilitate this process.

- *Passive diffusion.* This is the most important and most common mechanism of drug movement. If the drug concentration in the gastrointestinal tract is higher than its concentration in the bloodstream, then passive diffusion from areas of high to low concentration will drive the drug through the cell membrane into the circulation until an equilibrium with equal concentrations on either side is reached. No energy is expended during this process.
- *Facilitated diffusion.* This describes the transport of drugs of low lipid solubility across the cell membrane in combination with a carrier molecule. Again, it happens

in the presence of unequal concentrations and does not require energy.

- *Active transport.* Only drugs that closely resemble natural body substances can utilise this mechanism. Active transport works against a concentration gradient and requires a carrier molecule and the expenditure of energy.
- *Pinocytosis.* Intake into cells by this method, or 'cell-drinking', is not a common way for absorbing drugs. It requires energy and involves the cell membrane invaginating and engulfing a fluid-filled vesicle or sac.

Factors affecting absorption from the gastrointestinal tract

Anything that affects gastric motility and emptying will alter the rate of absorption, as will a range of other factors.

- *Gut motility.* Increases in gut motility decrease transit time and so the time available for drug absorption. Hypomotility may increase the amount of drug absorbed if contact with the gut epithelium is prolonged.
- *Gastric emptying.* Delayed gastric emptying will slow the delivery of drug to the intestine, thus reducing the absorption rate. If increased, it will increase drug absorption rate. The presence of gastric paresis, a complication of diabetes affecting the nerves of the stomach and causing delayed gastric emptying, is relevant here.

- *Surface area.*   Drug absorption is fastest in the small intestine because of the increased surface area provided by the villi.
- *Gut pH.*   The pH of the gastrointestinal tract varies along its length, which may affect different drugs in different ways. Optimal absorption of a drug may be dependent on a specific pH.
- *Blood flow.*   Faster absorption rates will occur in areas where blood supply is good; this is one reason why most absorption occurs in the small intestine, which has a very good blood supply.
- *Presence of food and fluid in the gastrointestinal tract.*   The presence of food in the gut may selectively increase or decrease drug absorption. For example, food increases the absorption of dicoumarol, while tetracycline absorption is reduced by the presence of dairy foods. Fluid taken with medication will aid dissolution of the drug and enhance its passage to the small intestine.
- *Antacids.*   The presence of antacids will increase absorption of basic drugs and decrease absorption of acidic ones.
- *Drug composition.*   This may affect absorption rates. For example, liquid preparations are more rapidly absorbed than solid ones. The presence of an enteric coating (e.g. in aspirin) may slow absorption, and lipid-soluble drugs are rapidly absorbed.

Absorption following parenteral administration

Intradermal drugs diffuse slowly from the injection site into local capillaries; for drugs administered subcutaneously, the process is a little faster. Because of the rich blood supply to muscles, absorption following an intramuscular injection is even quicker. The degree of tissue perfusion and condition of the injection site will influence the rate of drug absorption. Insulin is usually given subcutaneously. It will be absorbed slowly owing to the relatively poor blood supply in subcutaneous fat. However, if the patient accidentally injects into a muscle, the insulin will be absorbed rapidly, with a sudden drop in blood glucose and high risk of hypoglycaemia.

Absorption following topical administration

Absorption of drugs applied topically to mucous membranes and skin is lower than that of orally or parenterally administered drugs, although rates are higher if the skin is broken or the area is covered with an occlusive dressing. Rectal and sublingual absorption is usually rapid because of the vascularity of the mucosa. Absorption from instillation into the nose may lead to systemic as well as local effects, while inhalation into the lungs provides for extensive absorption. Minimal absorption will occur from instillation into the ears, but absorption from the eyes depends on whether a solution or ointment is administered. **Glucogel** (formerly known as Hypostop) is glucose suspended in a gel that can be rubbed into the inside of the cheeks in the treatment of mild to moderate hypoglycaemia (i.e. the patient is still conscious with a swallowing reflex).

Drug distribution

After absorption into the circulation, a drug is distributed: transported around the body to its target site. During this process, some molecules may be deposited at storage sites and others may be deposited and inactivated. A drug cannot exert its effect unless it reaches the target site in sufficient concentrations.

Factors affecting distribution rates

A range of factors affect distribution rates, and prescribers need to understand them to select appropriate formulations and administration routes.

- *Blood flow.* Distribution may depend on tissue perfusion. Organs that are highly vascularised, for example the heart, liver and kidneys, will rapidly acquire a drug, whereas concentrations in bone, fat, muscle and skin, for example, may take longer to rise. Skin and muscle have variable blood flows, and other factors such as activity levels and local tissue temperature may affect drug distribution to these areas. Some patients notice that absorption of insulin is faster if it is injected into abdominal fat than if injected into the thighs or buttocks. Also, during hot weather or sitting in a hot bath, insulin is absorbed from the skin more quickly than usual, which can cause hypoglycaemia

- *Plasma protein binding.* As most drugs that enter the circulation have low solubility, a proportion needs to be *bound*, or attached to, plasma proteins, usually albumin. If a drug is not bound to a plasma protein, it is said to be *free*. Drugs are inactive while bound to a plasma protein and have no pharmacological effect, as the size of the plasma proteins prevents them crossing cell membranes. Plasma binding is reversible as free molecules leave the circulation, more are released from plasma proteins so that an equilibrium between bound and free molecules is maintained. Binding tends to be non-specific and competitive: plasma proteins bind with many different drugs, and drugs will compete for binding sites on the plasma proteins. Displacement of one drug by another drug may have serious consequences, particularly if the therapeutic concentration of the drug is close to that which makes it toxic or ineffective. For example, warfarin can be displaced by tolbutamide, producing a risk of haemorrhage, while tolbutamide can be displaced by salicylates, producing a risk of hypoglycaemia.
- *Placental distribution barrier.* The chorionic villi enclose the fetal capillaries, which are separated from the maternal capillaries by a layer of trophoblastic cells. This layer acts as a barrier that allows the passage of lipid-soluble, non-ionised compounds from the mother

to the fetus, but prevents passage of substances with low lipid solubility. All women with diabetes who are planning a pregnancy should receive preconception counselling, and potential teratogenic drugs that cross the placental barrier should be discontinued. Women with type 2 diabetes will be changed to insulin instead of oral hypoglycaemic agents for the duration of the pregnancy.

- *Blood–brain barrier.*   Unlike capillaries elsewhere in the body, those in the central nervous system lack the channels between endothelial cells through which substances normally gain access to the extracellular fluid. This blood–brain barrier means that lipid-soluble drugs, for example diazepam, pass fairly readily into the central nervous system, but lipid-insoluble drugs have little or no effect.
- *Storage sites.*   Lipid-soluble drugs, for example anticoagulants, are stored in fat tissues, where they may remain until after administration has ceased. Calcium-containing structures such as bone and teeth can also accumulate calcium-binding drugs.

Drug metabolism

Drug metabolism – **biotransformation** – is the modification of the chemical composition of a drug, usually rendering it pharmacologically inactive. The products of this process – **metabolites** – are more highly ionised **(polar)** and less lipid-soluble than the original drug. They are, therefore, less likely to be reabsorbed across the cell membrane, promoting their excretion from the body. The metabolites of some drugs can also be pharmacologically active. Most drug metabolism occurs in the liver, catalysed by hepatic enzymes; it also occurs in the kidneys, intestinal mucosa, lungs, plasma and placenta.

There are two phases of metabolism, with some drugs undergoing both, and some one. In phase I, the drug is oxidised, reduced or hydrolysed to make it more polar. In phase II, drugs or phase I metabolites that are not sufficiently polar for excretion by the kidneys are made more **hydrophilic** ('water-liking') by conjugation (synthetic) reactions with endogenous liver compounds. The resulting conjugates are then readily excreted by the kidneys. If drugs are given repeatedly, their metabolism becomes more effective because of enzyme inductions; consequently, larger and larger doses are required to produce the same effect. This is known as **drug tolerance.** Adaptive changes at cell receptors may also lead to drug tolerance.

Factors affecting drug metabolism

Prescribers need a clear understanding of the various factors that can affect a patient's ability to metabolise drugs.

- *Genetic differences.*   Drug metabolism is controlled by genetically determined enzyme systems, leading to differences in responses. For example, some individuals show exaggerated and prolonged responses to drugs such as propranolol that undergo extensive hepatic metabolism.

- *Age.* In the elderly, first pass metabolism may be reduced, resulting in increased bioavailability. In addition, the delayed production and elimination of active metabolites may prolong drug action. Reduced doses may, therefore, be necessary for this group. In neonates, the enzyme systems responsible for conjugation are not fully effective and neonates may be at an increased risk of toxic effects of drugs. Glibenclamide is not recommended in the elderly as it stays in the system for longer than 24 hours as renal function falls. This can lead to prolonged and profound sulphonylurea-induced hypoglycaemia, which requires hospitalisation and intravenous glucose infusion until the drug has been excreted.
- *Disease processes.* Acute or chronic liver disease will affect metabolism if hepatocytes are destroyed. Reduced hepatic blood flow as a result of cardiac failure or shock may also reduce the rate of metabolism of drugs.

Drug excretion

Kidneys

Most drugs and metabolites are excreted by the kidneys, for example metformin. Small drug or metabolite molecules may be transported by glomerular filtration into the tubule, as long as they are not bound to plasma proteins. Active secretion of some drugs into the lumen of the nephron also occurs, in a process requiring membrane carriers and energy.

Several factors may affect the rate at which a drug is excreted by the kidneys: presence of kidney disease (e.g. renal failure), altered renal blood flow, urine pH, plasma concentration of the drug and molecular weight of the drug.

Bile

Several drugs and metabolites are secreted by the liver into bile. These then enter the duodenum via the common bile duct and move through the small intestine. Some drugs will be reabsorbed into the bloodstream and return to the liver by the enterohepatic circulation (Fig. 2.1). The drug then undergoes further metabolism or is secreted back into bile. This is referred to as enterohepatic cycling, and may extend the duration of action of a drug. Drugs secreted into bile will ultimately pass through the large intestine and be excreted in faeces.

Lungs

Anaesthetic gases and small amounts of alcohol undergo pulmonary excretion.

Breast milk

The glands that produce milk are surrounded by a network of capillaries, so drugs can pass from

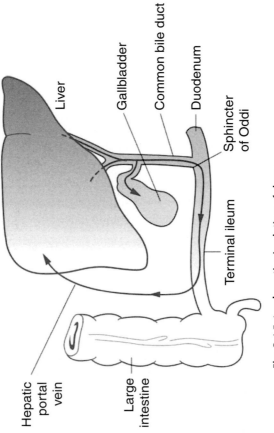

Liver

Gallbladder

Common bile duct

Duodenum

Sphincter
of Oddi

Terminal ileum

Hepatic
portal
vein

Large
intestine

Fig. 2.1 Enterohepatic circulation of drugs.

maternal blood into the breast milk. Although quantities may be very small, they can still have an effect because of babies' reduced ability to metabolise and excrete drugs.

Perspiration, saliva and tears

Lipid-soluble drugs can be excreted passively in perspiration, saliva and tears.

Half-lives and dosages

The processes of drug metabolism and drug excretion will ultimately determine the drug's **half-life**. This is the time taken for the concentration of drug in the blood to fall to 50% of its original value. Standard dosage intervals are based on half-life calculations to try to produce stable plasma drug concentrations, keeping the level of drug below toxic levels but above the minimum effective level. Achieving **steady state –** where the rate of elimination matches that of administration – takes longer for drugs with long half-lives. Sulphonylureas have long half-lives, for example that of glibenclamide is approximately 24 hours. Tolbutamide has a short half-life of approximately 6–8 hours. The half-lives of insulin analogues vary: short-acting analogues have half-lives of approximately 3–4 hours while long-acting analogues are approximately 24 hours.

Sometimes, a larger than normal dose of a drug is given because it is necessary to reach effective plasma levels quickly. This is called a **loading dose**. Once the required plasma level is reached, the normal recommended dose is given and continued at regular intervals to maintain a stable plasma level; this dose is called the **maintenance dose**.

When a drug with a narrow **therapeutic index** – ratio of toxic dose to its minimally effective dose – is used, its plasma levels are determined frequently (e.g. digoxin and lithium). Regular monitoring of drug plasma levels can also be used to assess a client's compliance with drug therapy.

Pharmacodynamics

Pharmacodynamics considers the effects of drugs on the body and their modes of action. All body functions are mediated by complex control systems involving enzymes, receptors on cell surfaces, carrier molecules and specific macromolecules, for example DNA. Most drugs act by interfering with these control systems at a molecular level. Drugs reach their cellular sites of action by the processes of absorption and distribution described and, once there, some work in a highly specific way, and some non-specifically.

Specific mechanisms of drug action

Interaction with receptors on the cell membrane

Receptors are protein molecules located either on the cell surface or intracellularly in the cytoplasm. Drugs have their effect at receptor sites by binding to them in the same way as the body's signalling molecules do, forming a drug–receptor complex. The drug and receptor must have complementary three-dimensional structures, in the same way that a key has a structure complementary to that of its lock (Fig. 2.2). Most drugs bind to more than one receptor and some drugs will combine with more than one type of receptor, but many drugs show selective activity at one particular receptor type e.g. glitazones bind to the gamma peroxisome proliferator activated receptors (PPAR-gamma).

Drugs bind to receptors to different extents, known as **affinities**, and the extent of their effects also varies. If a drug has an affinity for a receptor, and causes a specific response once bound, it is called an **agonist**. Morphine is an opioid agonist that binds to mu receptors in the central nervous system to depress the appreciation of pain. Drugs that bind to receptors and do not cause a response, blocking the receptors, are called **antagonists** as they prevent other drugs or messenger chemicals binding. **Competitive antagonists** compete with agonists for the receptor sites, thus inhibiting their action, but the extent of the effect depends on whether the agonist or antagonist occupies the most receptors. For example, naloxone is a competitive antagonist for mu receptors and may be used to treat opioid overdose. **Non-competitive antagonists** bind almost irreversibly to receptor sites, so agonists can have no effect. Drug–receptor binding is reversible and the response to the drug is gradually reduced as the drug molecules start to leave receptor sites.

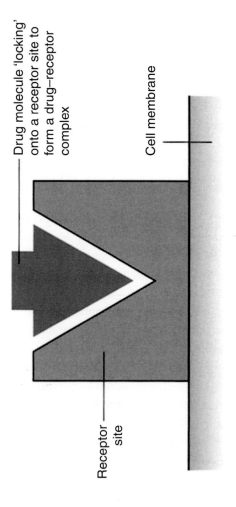

Drug molecule 'locking' onto a receptor site to form a drug–receptor complex

Receptor site

Cell membrane

Fig. 2.2 Complementry structure of drugs and their receptors.

Interference with ion passage through cell membranes

Ion channels are selective pores in the cell membrane that allow the movement of ions (for example, calcium and potassium) in and out of the cell, setting up electrical potential gradients across the membrane. Some drugs will block these channels, interfering with ion transport and altering physiological responses. Drugs working in this way include nifedipine, verapamil, lidocaine and sulphonylureas.

Enzyme inhibition or stimulation

Enzymes are proteins that act as biological catalysts, altering the rate of chemical reactions. Some drugs specifically interact with enzymes in a similar way to the formation of drug–receptor complexes. Sometimes, the drug resembles the enzyme's natural substrate and competes with it for the enzyme's binding sites. Sometimes, drugs bind irreversibly to the enzyme's active sites, rendering it ineffective. Drugs interacting with enzymes include aspirin, methotrexate and angiotensin-converting enzyme (ACE) inhibitors such as enalapril.

Incorporation into macromolecules

Some drugs are incorporated into larger molecules, interfering with their normal function. For example, when the anticancer drug 5-fluorouracil is incorporated into messenger RNA, taking the place of the molecule uracil, transcription is affected.

Interference with metabolic processes of microorganisms

Some drugs interfere with metabolic processes that are very specific or unique to microorganisms, thus either killing or inhibiting the activity of the microorganism. Penicillin disrupts bacterial cell wall formation while trimethoprim inhibits bacterial folic acid synthesis.

Non-specific mechanisms of drug action

Chemical alteration of the cellular environment

Drugs that do not alter specific cell function but alter the chemical environment around the cell can cause cellular responses or changes. Drugs that have this effect include osmotic diuretics (e.g. mannitol), osmotic laxatives (e.g. lactulose), and antacids (e.g. magnesium hydroxide).

Physical alteration of the cellular environment

Drugs can also alter the physical as opposed to the chemical environment around the cell, causing cellular responses or changes. Examples include docusate sodium, which lowers faecal surface tension, and many of the barrier preparations available, which protect the skin.

Unwanted effects of drug therapy

Most drugs have some unwanted effects, but those which are frequently prescribed, highly potent or that have a narrow therapeutic index are likely to increase the risk. There are several types of unwanted effect.

- *Adverse reactions/side-effects.* These will include any unwanted drug effects; examples are hypoglycaemia from sulphonlyureas, oedema with glitazones, diarrhoea from metformin.
- *Toxic effects.* These usually occur when too much drug has accumulated. It may be a result of an acutely high dose, chronic build up over time or increased sensitivity to the standard dose.
- *Drug allergies (hypersensitivities).* The body 'sees' the drug as an antigen and raises an immune response to it, either immediately or after a delay. Localised skin rashes in response to preservatives in insulin are seen, rarley, in diabetes. If this occurs, it may be necessary to change to another brand of insulin. Very rarely seen is anaphylactic shock following insulin injections.

Factors affecting a patient's response to a drug

Many individual factors will determine an individual's clinical response to a drug. Some of these have been discussed above: additional factors are discussed below. The prescriber should be fully aware of these factors and include them in the patient assessment before decisions are made about which drug to prescribe. All the factors should also be considered when monitoring prescribed or 'over-the-counter' drugs already used by the patient.

- *Age.*   Age can affect the ability to metabolise and excrete drugs, with the very young and the elderly in particular having problems. Because neonatal hepatic enzyme systems are not fully effective, drug metabolic rates are lower, leading to an increased risk of toxicity. In the elderly, delayed metabolism by the liver and a decline in renal function leads to a delay in excretion by the kidneys, which can prolong drug action. The longer-acting sulphonylurea glibenclamide increases the risk of hypoglycaemia in the elderly and so is not recommended. Complicated drug regimens may be difficult for the elderly to follow, which can mean incorrect doses are taken.
- *Body weight.*   The larger an individual, the greater the area the drug is distributed over, so the size of an individual affects drug concentrations. In addition, lipid-soluble drugs may be sequestered in fat stores and not available for use. Dosages of some drugs, therefore, need to be adjusted according to the patient's body weight (based on a dosage in milligrams per kilogram of body weight). All patients should have their weight recorded, and this should be reassessed regularly if drug treatment is long term. Generally, the larger the patient, the larger the dose of insulin required. Patients who lose weight will need to reduce their insulin dose; some with type 2 diabetes may even be able to discontinue their insulin injections altogether.
- *Pregnancy and lactation.*   Lipid-soluble, non-ionised drugs in the free state will cross the placenta (examples

include opiates and warfarin). Some drugs cause fetal malformation. Drugs transferred via breast milk can also have adverse effects on the baby (e.g. sedatives, anticonvulsants and caffeine). If possible, a full drug history should be obtained before conception, and at least on confirmation of pregnancy. Pregnant women, or those planning a pregnancy, should be advised not to take medication without consulting a physician, pharmacist, midwife or nurse. Preconception counselling, particularly for young women with type 2 diabetes and planning a pregnancy, should be provided. Often these women are taking an ACE inhibitor for hypertension and statins for dyslipidaemia.

- *Nutritional status.* Malnutrition can alter drug distribution and metabolism. Inadequate dietary protein may affect enzyme activity and slow the metabolism of drugs; reductions in plasma protein levels may increase amounts of available free drug, and reduced body fat stores will mean lower sequestering of the drug in fat. Normal doses in the severely malnourished may lead to toxicity. Consequently, nutritional assessment of patients is essential and malnutrition should be managed accordingly.

- *Food–drug interactions.* The presence of food may affect drug absorption. For example, orange juice (which contains vitamin C) will enhance the absorption of iron sulphate, but dairy produce reduces the absorption of tetracycline. Monoamine oxidase inhibitors must not be taken with foods rich in tyramine (including cheese, meat yeast extracts, some types of alcoholic drink) because of possible toxic effects, such as a sudden hypertensive crisis. Grapefruit should not be eaten by patients taking statins as the fruit can interfere with statin metabolism in the liver. Prescribers should have some knowledge of common food–drug interactions and drug administration may need to be timed in relation to mealtimes.

- *Disease processes.* Altered functioning of many body systems will affect a client's response to a drug: a few examples are given here.
  - Changes in gut motility and, therefore, transit time may affect absorption rates, so diarrhoea and vomiting lower absorption. Loss of absorptive surface in the small intestine, as occurs in Crohn's disease, will also affect absorption.
  - Hepatic disease (e.g. hepatitis, cirrhosis and liver failure) will reduce drug metabolism and lead to a gradual accumulation of drugs and risk of toxicity.
  - Renal disease (e.g. acute and chronic renal failure) will reduce excretion of drugs and may lead to accumulation; For example metformin can provoke lactic acidosis in patients with renal impairment.
  - Circulatory diseases (e.g. heart failure and peripheral vascular disease) will reduce distribution and transport of drugs.
- *Mental and emotional factors.* Compliance with a drug regimen can be affected by many varied factors, including confusion, amnesia, identified mental illness,

stress and bereavement. Resulting inadequate or excessive use of medication can render treatment unsuccessful or produce serious adverse effects. The prescriber must consider these issues in the patient assessment.

- *Genetic and ethnic factors.* Genetic variations lead to differences in patients' abilities to metabolise drugs. For example, some individuals possess an atypical form of the enzyme pseudocholinesterase. When these individuals are given the muscle relaxant suxamethonium, prolonged paralysis occurs and recovery from the drug takes longer. Different races of people are also known to dispose of drugs at different rates.

FURTHER READING

Downie G. and Mackenzie J. (1999) *Pharmacology and Drug Management for Nurses*, 2nd edn. Edinburgh: Churchill Livingstone.

Galbraith A., Bullock S., Manias E., Richards A. and Hunt B. (1999) *Fundamentals of Pharmacology: A Text for Nurses and Health Professionals*. Singapore: Addison Wesley Longman.

Pinnell N. L. (1996) *Nursing Pharmacology*. Philadelphia, PA: W. B. Saunders.

Rang H. P., Dale M. M., Ritter J. M. and Moore P.K. (2003) *Pharmacology*, 5th edn. Edinburgh: Churchill Livingstone.

Springhouse (2004) *Clinical Pharmacology Made Incredibly Easy!* 2nd edn. Springhouse, PA: Springhouse Corporation.

Trounce J. R. and Gould D. (2000) *Clinical Pharmacology for Nurses*, 16th edn. Edinburgh: Churchill Livingstone.

Chapter 3

Normal blood glucose regulation and diabetes

Blood glucose levels in the individual without diabetes remain remarkably stable, approximately between 4 and 7 mmol/l, even if the individual fasts for several hours or consumes a large sugary meal. This level is maintained by a relationship between insulin, which lowers blood glucose, and the counter-regulatory hormones (primarily glucagon), which cause a rise in blood glucose (Table 3.1). The efficiency of this system is often not appreciated until the prescriber tries to support the patient with diabetes to mimic these same effects and achieve near normoglycaemia with the various manufactured insulins available!

Insulin is produced by the beta cells in the islets of Langerhans, embedded in the pancreas gland (which also produces pancreatic digestive juices, a function that is not affected in diabetes). After a carbohydrate load in the gut following eating, starch and sugars are broken down into glucose by digestive juices. Glucose is then absorbed from the gut into the blood circulation. Receptors in the beta cells monitor the prevailing blood glucose. In the individual without diabetes, the resulting rise in blood glucose after a meal stimulates the beta cells to produce

Table 3.1 The main hormones affecting blood glucose concentrations

	Insulin	Glucagon
Actions	Facilitates transport of glucose across cell membranes (to be converted to energy)	Stimulates breakdown of liver glycogen back to glucose (glucogenolysis)
	Facilitates the conversion of glucose to glycogen (in liver and muscles)	Stimulates the liver to make glucose from other substances (gluconeogenesis)
	Prevents the breakdown of stored glycogen back to glucose (glygenolysis) by inhibiting production of glucagon	
	Prevents the production of glucose from other substances by the liver (gluconeogenesis) by inhibiting production of glucagon	
Release	From pancreatic beta cells, stimulated by rising levels of blood glucose	From pancreatic alpha cells, stimulated by low levels of insulin and blood glucose

a burst of insulin, which prevents blood glucose from rising much above 7 mmol/l. As the blood glucose falls to normal as feeding finishes, beta cell stimulation is reduced and insulin production also falls in response.

During periods of fasting, low blood glucose concentrations result in minimal stimulation of the beta cells, so production of insulin is low. Insulin has an inhibitory effect on glucose output by the liver, by suppressing glycogenolysis (breakdown of glycogen stores) and gluconeogenesis (production of glucose from other substrates). Low levels of circulating insulin means less suppression of these processes, which allows blood glucose levels to rise as glucose is released from the liver. This is the mechanism that stops blood glucose from falling too low, even during periods of fasting. The rising blood glucose then stimulates the beta cells to produce insulin again, which lowers blood glucose, maintaining a fasting blood glucose of around 3.5 to 6 mmol/l in the individual without diabetes (Fig. 3.1).

Diabetes

The content of this book relates to the two main types of diabetes: type 1 and type 2. Although patients are commonly assigned to one of the two types, there may be a continuum between the two, as some patients may not present with the classical signs or symptoms of either type. Also, with the increase in obesity in children, type 2 diabetes is now occurring in this age group, whereas before the mid-1990s, a child presenting with diabetes was almost always diagnosed with type 1 diabetes. Type 1 diabetes also occasionally presents in people aged over 40, which typically is the age at which type 2 diabetes develops. Any patient, therefore, who presents with hyperglycaemia, is unwell and with significant weight loss should be assumed

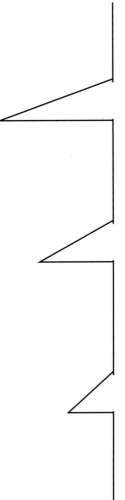

Fig. 3.1 Insulin production in the non-diabetic state, showing basal (or background) insulin maintaining normal fasting blood glucose and boluses (or mealtime spikes) preventing the blood glucose from rising too high after a carbohydrate load.

to potentially have type 1 diabetes, and monitored regularly, until proved otherwise, no matter what age they are.

Gestational diabetes, which is a condition of glucose intolerance that presents during pregnancy, and the rarer types of diabetes such as mature-onset diabetes in the young (MODY), are not discussed here as they are generally managed in specialist diabetes units.

Diabetes is becoming very common worldwide. In the UK, it was estimated in 1989 that there were 1.3 million people living with the condition. This figure was predicted to rise to 3.1 million by 2010 (Amos *et al.*, 1997). This epidemic is caused by the increase in the number of people developing type 2 diabetes and is closely related to the increasing number of people who are overweight or obese. It has serious implications for the use of NHS resources as diabetes is costly, estimated in 2001 as consuming around 5–10% of the total NHS budget (DoH, 2001). About 40% of this expenditure is used in the management of preventable complications of diabetes (Baxter *et al.*, 2000). All patients with diabetes, whether type 1 or type 2, are at risk of developing diabetic complications. These include microvascular diseases (retinopathy, neuropathy, and nephropathy) and macrovascular diseases (myocardial infarction, angina, stroke and peripheral vascular disease). Successful management of blood glucose, blood pressure, lipids and other risk factors reduces the risk of diabetes complications (Stratton *et al.*, 2000) (Table 3.2).

Table 3.2 The evidence-base for reducing diabetes complications in types 1 and 2 diabetes

Trials	Trial results
Type 1	
Diabetes Control and Complications Trial Research Group, 1993	This trial involved 1441 patients with type 1 diabetes, of which 726 had no retinopathy and 715 had mild retinopathy. They were assigned to (i) intensive insulin therapy using an insulin pump or to three or four daily insulin injections and frequent blood glucose monitoring and support, or (ii) to conventional therapy (which at the time was once or twice daily insulin injections). The results showed that intensive insulin therapy delayed the onset and slowed the progression of retinopathy, nephropathy and neuropathy
Type 2	
UK Prospective Diabetes Study (UKPDS) Group, 1998	The UKPDS 33 trial involved 3867 people with newly diagnosed type 2 diabetes, treated with insulin, chlorpropamide, glibenclamide or glipizide. It demonstrated that intensive treatment with either sulphonylureas or insulin substantially reduced the risk of microvascular but not macrovascular complications
Turner *et al.*, 1998	In the UK Prospective Diabetes Study (UKPDS) 38, 1148 hypertensive patients with type 2 diabetes were allocated to either tight blood pressure control or less tight control. Drugs used were captopril and atenolol. This trial demonstrated that fatal and non-fatal cardiovascular complications and deterioration in visual acuity are reduced by tight control of blood pressure compared with less tight control. It also showed that more than one antihypertensive agent may be required

Type 1 diabetes

Type 1 diabetes (previously known as insulin-dependent diabetes (IDDM) or juvenile-onset diabetes) makes up approximately 20% of the diabetic population and usually presents in children and young adults. It is caused by an autoimmune-mediated destruction of the insulin-producing beta cells in the pancreas, eventually causing a complete lack of insulin. Treatment is always, therefore, insulin-replacement therapy.

The onset is usually sudden, with a short history of a few weeks of marked weight loss, thirst, polyuria and lethargy. As insulin production falls, blood glucose concentrations rise. This causes an osmotic diuresis (hence the polyuria), which causes dehydration (resulting in thirst). Loss of calories (glucose) in the urine contributes to weight loss. Glucose is less able to cross cell membranes to be converted into energy, causing exhaustion. Alternative energy pathways involving fat metabolism are used instead by the body. This results in the production of ketones, an alternative energy source, which can be detected in the urine, blood and on the breath. Unfortunately, as these accumulate, they reduce the pH of the blood, leading to acidosis. Without treatment with insulin, this alternative energy production pathway is used predominantly, and diabetic ketoacidosis develops, with the patient presenting as a medical emergency: unconscious, dehydrated and acidotic. This once common presentation of type 1 diabetes is becoming less common as public awareness of the signs and symptoms of diabetes has increased. The classic osmotic symptoms with loss of weight will often prompt someone to consider that they may have diabetes.

As the beta cells have been destroyed, insulin-replacement therapy is currently the only treatment option. Oral hypoglycaemic agents are completely ineffective in these patients as they work by either stimulating beta cells to produce more insulin or improving the body's sensitivity to insulin (so will not work if there are no beta cells or insulin available). In the absence of insulin, blood glucose levels rise as there is no block on the liver releasing glucose, even if the patient is not eating. Without treatment with insulin, this leads to ketoacidosis and eventually death. People with type 1 diabetes are, therefore, completely dependent on insulin: if they stop it or omit a dose, blood glucose will rise, even if they are not eating anything. The rule with type 1 patients is NEVER STOP INSULIN.

Type 2 diabetes

Type 2 diabetes (previously known as non-insulin-dependent diabetes (NIDDM) or mature-onset diabetes) is usually associated with obesity and lack of physical activity, and is the main cause of the diabetes epidemic seen nationally and worldwide, mirroring the increasing trends of these aspects of westernised lifestyle.
Patients are usually older than 30 years but type 2 diabetes is now being diagnosed in some very overweight

children. People who are at risk of developing the condition include those over 40, those of South Asian or Afro-Caribbean descent, those who are overweight, those who have a family history of diabetes, and those women who have had gestational diabetes or a large baby (over 4 kg) in the past.

Type 2 diabetes is a complex condition and is a manifestation of the **metabolic syndrome**. This includes hypertension, dyslipidaemia, central obesity, clotting abnormalities and inadequately compensated insulin resistance (Table 3.3). Patients usually require medication to address most or all of these factors, and are prescribed a large number of drugs, with a concomitantly large number of tablets to take. Unfortunately, there is evidence that many patients do not take these tablets as prescribed (Donnan *et al.*, 2002).

Type 2 diabetes is progressive. For years before diagnosis, sensitivity to insulin action by the tissues decreases (insulin resistance) and there is a compensatory increase in insulin production by the beta cells. (Put simply: if insulin action is only half as effective as normal, so long as the beta cells can produce twice as much insulin, then blood glucose levels will remain within the normal range.) Eventually however, this compensation becomes inadequate as the beta cells start to fail. The typical treatment history of someone with type 2 diabetes progresses from diet and lifestyle modification alone, then oral hypoglycaemic agents, and eventually to insulin therapy, a history reflecting

Table 3.3 The characteristics of the metabolic syndrome as defined by the International Diabetes Federation (2005)

Characteristic	Definition
Central obesity	Waist > 94 cm in men (90 cm in Asian men); > 80 cm in women
Plus at least two of the following:	
Raised blood pressure	$> 130/85$ or treatment of previously diagnosed hypertension
Raised HDL cholesterol	> 1.03 mmol/l in men, > 1.29 mmol/l in women, or specific treatment for this lipid abnormality
Raised triglycerides	> 1.7 mmol/l or specific treatment for this lipid abnormality
Raised fasting blood glucose	5.6. mmol/l or greater (or previously diagnosed type 2 diabetes) (currently 6.1 mmol/l or higher is still the level at which impaired fasting glycaemia is diagnosed in the UK)

HDL, high density lipoprotein.

progression from insulin resistance to beta cell failure (Wright *et al.*, 2002).

Initially, if lifestyle changes alone are ineffective, oral agents are chosen to address insulin resistance in the early stages of type 2 diabetes (such as metformin and glitazones). As beta cell failure progresses, insulin secretagogues may be used to stimulate insulin production. Eventually, however, the beta cells cannot produce sufficient insulin to compensate for the insulin resistance and insulin therapy is added to supplement the patient's own insulin production. These patients do not become type 1 diabetics; they continue to have type 2 diabetes, managed with insulin therapy.

The development of type 2 diabetes is insidious, with years of gradually increasing insulin resistance and glucose intolerance with very few signs and symptoms. There may be tiredness, nocturia, dry mouth and infections such as balanitis or vaginal thrush. Many patients do not have weight loss. Some patients may not notice any symptoms at all and may be diagnosed through opportunistic screening. However, some may present with diabetes complications such as myocardial infarction, gangrene or visual loss. Many patients presenting with newly diagnosed diabetes already have diabetic damage as they have had the condition for years without realising (UK Prospective Diabetes Study, 1998).

Making the diagnosis

Diabetes is defined as a condition characterised by a chronically raised plasma glucose concentration (hyperglycaemia) caused by a complete or relative lack of maintenance of blood glucose within normal levels by the hormone insulin (Watkins, 1998). Despite this very clear definition, diagnosing diabetes may not be simple. Being diagnosed with diabetes has major implications for that person's way of life, so it is essential that there is no doubt about the diagnosis. The World Health

Table 3.4 World Health Organization 1999 classification of glucose states

Classification	Fasting blood glucose (mmol/l)	Blood glucose 2 hours after a 75 g glucose load (mmol/l)
Non-diabetic	≤ 6.0	< 7.8
Impaired fasting glycaemia	6.1–6.9	< 7.8
Impaired glucose tolerance	< 7.0	7.8–11.0
Diabetes	≥ 7.0	≥ 11.1

Organization has provided clear criteria for establishing the presence of diabetes and impaired glucose tolerance (Table 3.4).

Diagnosis of type 1 diabetes is usually clear cut. A short history of osmotic symptoms with significant weight loss and with a venous sample in the diagnostic range will confirm the diagnosis. Ketones may not be present in the urine or blood in significant amounts if the condition is identified early, but if present, this usually confirms that the patient has type 1 rather than type 2 diabetes.

The natural history of type 2 diabetes includes various stages of glucose intolerance during the development of the condition. If the patient has symptoms plus one abnormal venous blood glucose result (i.e. their fasting venous blood glucose is 7 mmol/l or higher, or a random venous sample is 11.1 mmol/l or higher), a definite diagnosis can be made. If the patient has no symptoms, then two abnormal venous samples taken on different days are required to diagnose diabetes.

In the absence of diabetes, the normal fasting venous blood glucose is 6.0 mmol/l or less and it does not rise above 7.7 mmol/l after a 75 g glucose load. Results higher than these, therefore, indicate abnormal blood glucose levels.

If the fasting blood glucose is between 6.1 and 6.9 mmol/l, then a diagnosis of **impaired fasting glycaemia** (IFG) is made. People with this condition have an increased risk of developing diabetes in the future. A formal oral glucose tolerance test (OGTT) should be performed to exclude the diagnosis of diabetes. If the results of the OGTT show the fasting blood glucose is less than 7 mmol/l and the value 2 hours after a glucose load is between 7.8 and 11.0 mmol/l, then a diagnosis of **impaired glucose tolerance** (IGT) is made. Although neither IGT nor IFG is associated with the microvascular complications seen in diabetes, they are associated with increased risk of cardiovascular disease, particularly IGT.

REFERENCES

Amos A. F., McCarty D. J. and Zimmet P. (1997) The rising global burden of diabetes and its complications: estimates and projections to the year 2010. *Diabetic Medicine* **14**(Suppl. 5): S1–S85.

Baxter H., Bottomley J., Burns E. *et al.* (2000) CODE-2 UK. The annual direct costs of care for people with type 2 diabetes in Great Britain. *Diabetic Medicine* **17**(Suppl. 1): 13.

Diabetes Control and Complications Trial Research Group (1993) The effect of intensive treatment of diabetes on the development and progression of long-term complications in insulin-dependent diabetes mellitus. *New England Journal of Medicine* **329**: 977–86.

DoH (2001) *National Service Framework for Diabetes: Standards.* London: The Stationery Office.

Donnan P. T., MacDonald T. M. and Morris A. D. (2002) Adherence to prescribed oral hypoglycaemic medication in a population of patients with type 2 diabetes: a retrospective cohort study. *Diabetes Medicine* **19**: 279–84.

International Diabetes Federation (2005) *The IDF Consensus Worldwide Definition of the Metabolic Syndrome.* Brussels: International Diabetes Federation. Available at www.idf.org/webdata/docs/IDF/Metasyndrome/definition.pdf,2005 (January accessed 26 2007).

Stratton I. M., Adler A. I. and Andrew H. (2000) Association of glycaemia with macrovascular and microvascular complications of type 2 diabetes (UKPDS 35): prospective observational study. *British Medical Journal* **321**: 405–12.

Turner R., Holman R., Stratton I., for the UK Prospective Diabetes Study (UKPDS) Group (1998) Tight blood pressure control and risk of macrovascular and microvascular complications in type 2 diabetes: UKPDS 38. *British Medical Journal* **317**: 703–13.

UK Prospective Diabetes Study (UKPDS) Group (1998) Intensive blood-glucose control with sulphonylureas or insulin compared with conventional treatment and risk of complications in patients with type 2 diabetes (UKPDS 33). *Lancet* **352**: 837–53.

Watkins P. (1998) *ABC of Diabetes*. London: BMJ Publishing.

World Health Organization (1999) *Definition, Diagnosis and Classification of Diabetes Mellitus and its Complications*. Part 1. *Diagnosis and Classification of Diabetes Mellitus*. Geneva: World Health Organization.

Wright A., Burden A. C., Paisley R. B., Cull C. A. and Holman R. R. (2002) Sulfonyl inadequacy: efficacy of addition of insulin over 6 years in patients with type 2 diabetes in the UK Prospective Diabetes Study (UKPDS 57). *Diabetes Care* **25**: 330–6.

Chapter 4

Supporting lifestyle changes and patient empowerment

Three approaches are important for people with diabetes:

- weight management
- smoking cessation
- self-monitoring of glucose levels.

Whether their diabetes is managed with tablets or insulin or no medication, people with diabetes need to adopt a healthy eating plan, increase daily physical activity and avoid damaging lifestyle behaviours. This will help them to achieve control of blood glucose, cholesterol, blood pressure and weight. There is clear evidence for both type 1 diabetes (Diabetes Control and Complications Trial, 1993) and type 2 diabetes (UK Prospective Diabetes Study, 1998) that keeping good control of these factors reduces the risk of developing microvascular and macrovascular diabetes complications. Standard 3 of the National Service Framework for Diabetes (DoH, 2001 (Box 4.1)) and the guidelines for structured education from the National Institute of Health and Clinical Effectiveness (NICE guidance, 2003) make recommendations for informing and empowering people with diabetes to make changes to adopt a healthy lifestyle.

Box 4.1 Standard 3 of the National Service Framework for Diabetes

All children, young people and adults with diabetes will receive a service which encourages partnership in decision-making, supports them in managing their diabetes and helps them to adopt a healthy lifestyle. This will be reflected in an agreed and shared care plan in an appropriate format and language. Where appropriate, parents and carers should be fully engaged in this process.

Assessment of the readiness for making changes is essential. For example, a simple Likert scale can be used when asking, on a scale of 1 to 10, how important is it to you to make this change (where 0 is not important and 10 is very important), and also on a scale of 1 to 10, how confident do you feel that you are able to make the change (where 0 is not at all confident and 10 is very confident). This helps patients to identify their priorities for behaviour change, any barriers that may prevent them achieving their aim, and to set realistic goals. However, even if they are ready to make changes and despite provision of information and support, many patients need pharmacological intervention to support weight loss and giving up smoking.

Weight management

Weight management, healthy eating and regular physical activity are essential foundations for anyone with diabetes to reduce risk of cardiovascular disease and to control blood glucose, to which oral hypoglycaemic agents and/or insulin are added (i.e. a healthy lifestyle is not an optional extra!). Weight management is a particular issue for overweight people with type 2 diabetes, as excess weight is a significant cause of insulin resistance. In these patients, insulin production is often more than adequate in the early stages of diabetes but the effects of insulin resistance mean that the beta cells have to produce relatively large amounts of insulin to overcome the poor sensitivity to the effects of insulin.

Losing weight often improves the body's sensitivity to the effects of insulin (i.e. reduces insulin resistance) and may delay the progression onto oral hypoglycaemic agents and insulin. If patients are obese and unable to lose sufficient weight with diet alone, then anti-obesity agents to facilitate weight loss may be the most suitable first-line treatment in glycaemic management (although these agents are not specifically licensed as hypoglycaemic agents). In patients with impaired glucose tolerance, losing weight may delay or even prevent the progression to diabetes (Diabetes Prevention Program Research Group, 2002).

There are three possible pharmacological agents that may be appropriate to support weight loss. However, patients should be clear that drugs are in addition to lifestyle intervention, not instead of, and they are not a stand-alone treatment for obesity. A combination of strategies incorporating diet, regular physical activity and behavioural approaches with one of these agents is more likely to be successful than the drug alone. Clear realistic goals for the treatment should be agreed with the patient:

1. Prevent further weight gain
2. Promote a clinically significant but realistic weight loss (ideally 5–10%)
3. Support long-term weight maintenance
4. Drugs should be discontinued if there is not at least 5% body weight loss from starting the medication within an agreed time frame.

Orlistat (Xenical)

Orlistat is a pancreatic lipase inhibitor that prevents the breakdown of dietary fat to fatty acids and glycerol, decreasing fat absorption by up to 30% and causing an increase in the fat content of faeces (thus removing potential calories from the body). Orlistat is taken with food, 120 mg three times a day. It can increase weight loss by approximately 2–4 kg more over a year than is achieved by calorie restriction alone.

Orlistat is recommended for patients with a body mass index (BMI) > 30, or > 28 in the presence of other risk factors such as type 2 diabetes. Patients should start with 120 mg with their main meal and then titrate up to 120 mg three times a day. It can be continued if there has been a weight loss of 5% or greater of total body weight after three months and > 10% after six months. It should not be continued for more than two years.

Side-effects include abdominal cramps, excessive flatus production and diarrhoea, sometimes with faecal incontinence, oily spotting and intestinal borborymi (rumbling). Diarrhoea is particularly a problem if the patient continues to eat a diet with a high fat content (and, therefore, this medication can be an important education tool for patients who incorrectly feel they are following a healthy diet). A support system is available for patients using orlistat, which includes information and telephone calls to increase motivation. This can have a significant impact on the effectiveness of the medication. Patients should be encouraged to contact the service on 0800 731 7138 or visit the website www.xenicalmap.co.uk.

Excretion.   It is excreted via the faeces as very little is absorbed from the gut.

Contraindications.   It should not be used in patients with malabsorption problems or cholestasis, or during pregnancy and breast-feeding.

Cautions.   There may be a decreased absorption of the contraceptive pill. Patients may need a supplement of fat-soluble vitamins, taken between meals.

Sibutramine (Reductil)

Sibutramine acts by inhibiting the reuptake of the neurotransmitters noradrenaline and serotonin from receptor sites in the hypothalamus. This has two effects. It enhances satiety by serotonin stimulation of the $5HT_{2A}$ and $5HT_{2C}$ receptors. It may also increase energy expenditure by increasing sympathetic stimulation of thermogenesis. It enhances satiety, can reduce waist circumference (i.e. visceral fat), decrease plasma triglycerides and very low density lipoprotein (VLDL) cholesterol, but cause an increase in protective high density lipoprotein (HDL) cholesterol. It will reduce weight by 2–4 kg more than low calorie diet alone over a year, and it is recommended for people with a BMI > 30, or > 27 in the presence of other risk factors such as type 2 diabetes.

Sibutramine is taken orally and is well absorbed. It does not have any addictive or antidepressant properties. The initial dose is 10 mg daily (but can be increased to 15 mg daily after four weeks) for a maximum of a year.

Excretion.   Active metabolites are deactivated by the liver and excreted in the urine and faeces.

Side-effects.   These include dry mouth, anxiety, constipation and insomnia.

Contraindications.   As sibutramine can increase heart rate and blood pressure (through sympathetic activity), it is contraindicated if the patient has ischaemic heart disease, cardiac failure, arrhythmias or uncontrolled hypertension. It should not be used with monoamine oxidase inhibitors or tryptophan, in patients with a history of major eating disorders or psychiatric illness, and during pregnancy or breast-feeding.

Monitoring.   Pulse rate and blood pressure should be checked regularly (every two weeks for first three months, then monthly for the next three months, and then every three months). Interactions with drugs that are metabolised by one of the P450 isoenzymes can occur.

Rimonabant (Accomplia)

Rimonabant has just recently been licensed and guidelines for its use were being developed by NICE at the time of publication of this book. It works by suppressing appetite by selectively blocking the cannabinoid-1 (CB1) receptor in the endocannabinoid system in the brain. It is licensed for use as an adjunct to diet and exercise for patients with a BMI of > 27 and diabetes (or BMI > 30 if no diabetes). The 20 mg tablet should be taken daily before breakfast, in combination with a healthy, mildly reduced calorie diet. A patient support programme can be accessed through www.itswhatyougain.com.

Side-effects.   These include depressive symptoms and mood disorders, and so it should not be used by patients with uncontrolled serious psychiatric disorders or those taking antidepressants. Other common side-effects include nausea (about 10% of patients), anxiety, insomnia and mood alterations.

Contraindications.   Psychiatric disorders, severe renal impairment, pregnancy and breast-feeding are all contraindications.

Interactions.   Inhibitors of CYP3A4 (e.g. ketoconazole, ritonavir) will increase plasma levels of rimonabant and CYP3A4 inducers (e.g. phenytoin, carbamazepine, St John's wort) will lower plasma concentrations.

Patients requiring specialist help

NICE recommend that use of bariatric surgery should be considered in patients with a BMI of > 35 if other interventions are not successful.

Smoking cessation

People with diabetes, especially type 2 diabetes, have a high risk of cardiovascular and peripheral vascular disease. Smoking cigarettes is also a huge risk factor for these conditions, as well as increasing risk of cancers and chronic bronchitis (tar and other irritants rather than nicotine), and having harmful effects in pregnancy. The management of diabetes is focused on reducing risk of complications and reducing or eliminating risk factors: smoking is a significant risk factor. There is a strong correlation between stroke, diabetic gangrene, coronary heart disease, peripheral vascular disease and smoking. One study suggested that patients with type 2 diabetes have the same risk of having a myocardial infarction as someone without diabetes who has already had a myocardial infarction (Haffner *et al.*, 1998). Support for patients with diabetes and who smoke, and who want to stop, is, therefore, extremely important.

There are three agents used to treat nicotine dependence: nicotine replacement therapy, bupropion and varenicline. Guidelines from NICE recommend that smoking cessation treatments should only be prescribed when a patient wants to stop smoking and commits to a target stop date. One therapy only should be used at a time, as there is insufficient evidence to recommend the use of two therapies together. The most successful smoking-cure clinics use a combination of psychological and pharmacological interventions, and still only achieve a success rate of about 25% (i.e. percentage of patients still not smoking after a year). If the patient fails to stop smoking, smoking cessation therapy should not normally be prescribed for a further six months.

Nicotine replacement therapy

Nicotine replacement therapy works by relieving the psychological and physical withdrawal syndrome. It comes in a variety of forms including chewing gum, lozenges, sublingual tablets, nasal spray and inhalator and needs to be taken several times a day as nicotine is relatively shortacting. Alternatively, it can be prescribed as transdermal patches, which are replaced daily initially. The use of counselling and supportive therapy is essential: it has been demonstrated in double-blind trials that nicotine alone is no more effective than placebo. It should, therefore, only be prescribed by trained smoking counsellors or through a smoking cessation support programme. These are available through the NHS stop-smoking services, pharmacists, practice nurses or smoking cessation programmes delivered through Primary Care Trusts by appropriately trained educators (NICE Technology Appraisal No. 39).

Contraindications.   As nicotine can cause coronary spasm, it should not be used in patients with heart disease or recent myocardial infarction.

Side-effects.   Nicotine can cause various side-effects including nausea, gastrointestinal cramps, cough, headache, insomnia and muscle spasm. The patches can cause local irritation and itching.

Bupropion

Bupropion is an antidepressant but appears to be as effective in supporting smoking cessation as nicotine replacement therapy, even in people who are not depressed. It probably works by inhibiting the reuptake of dopamine and noradrenaline, increasing the activity of these transmitters in areas of the brain associated with symptoms of withdrawal and dependence. One of these is the nucleus accumbens (which is involved with the 'reward pathway'). It, therefore, reduces the craving and withdrawal symptoms when stopping smoking.

Contraindications.   This agent should be avoided in patients with a history of seizures, tumour of the central nervous system, bipolar disorder and eating disorders.

Caution.   Blood pressure should be monitored before and during treatment.

Side-effects.   Bupropion can cause insomnia, headache, dry mouth and taste disorders but it has a lower side-effect risk than nicotine replacement therapy.

Varenicline

Varenicline is awaiting NICE guidance for its use, due out during the summer of 2007, but it is likely to be recommended as an option for smoking cessation and to be prescribed only as part of a programme of behavioural support. It is an oral selective partial agonist of nicotinic receptors that is designed to block the rewards for, and reduce the cravings for, cigarette smoking. Its use with people with diabetes has not been investigated.

Side-effects.   These include nausea, insomnia, abnormal dreams and headaches. It is more costly than nicotine replacement or bupropion.

Self-monitoring

Diabetes is a life-long condition and the development of self-management skills is essential for the successful management of the condition. The increasing number of people developing diabetes has also necessitated a move away from the prescriptive paternalistic care practised by healthcare professionals in the past, to empowering patients to make decisions about adjusting insulin doses etc. The National Service Framework for Diabetes third standard (out of 12) is devoted to the education and empowerment of people with diabetes (Box 4.1). Self-monitoring of blood or urine glucose and ketone levels can provide patients with information with which to make informed decisions about the management of their glucose control.

Home blood glucose monitoring consumes a large amount of NHS resources, both in direct cost of the strips required for testing, and healthcare professional time in training. There is very little argument about its value for patients using insulin therapy, but the evidence for its usefulness is sparse for patients with type 2 diabetes managed on lifestyle alone or oral therapies. In fact, self-monitoring of blood glucose can increase distress, worry and depressive symptoms for people not using insulin (Franciosi *et al.*, 2001).

Some authorities have limited the prescribing of blood testing strips to insulin users only. However, the tests provide feedback to patients about how well their blood glucose is controlled, and their use informs them how any intervention that they make has affected their levels (e.g. the effect of exercise). This feedback can be an effective motivator to make and maintain changes to a healthier lifestyle. The value of monitoring, how often and the best times to test should be negotiated with patients when discussing their diabetes management plan, usually at the diabetes annual review. NICE recommend self-monitoring should not be considered as a stand-alone intervention but taught if the need/purpose is clear and agreed with the patient. It can form an important part of self-care.

Monitoring glucose levels

Urine glucose testing

The underlying principle of testing for the presence of glucose in a urine sample is that if blood glucose has exceeded the renal threshold for glucose (about 10 mmol/l in most people) since the last time the patient passed urine, then glucose will appear in the urine. If blood glucose has remained below the glucose renal threshold, then the urine sample will be negative for glucose. The ideal result, therefore, should be always negative.

The strips are relatively low in cost compared with blood glucose-monitoring strips (between about £2.50 and £3.00 for 50 urine tests) and have the advantage that they do not involve the use of a meter and are non-invasive and pain free. However, this assumes that the patient has a normal renal threshold. Unfortunately, some patients may have quite high blood glucose levels yet still have negative urine glucose levels as their renal thresholds are well into double figures. Conversely, if the patient has an abnormally low renal threshold, then they will have false-positive urine glucose results: glucose will appear in the urine despite having normal blood glucose levels. As the test shows if glucose has escaped into the urine since the patient last passed urine, a positive test does not inform the patient about blood glucose concentration at the time of the test. It is possible for the patient to be hypoglycaemic yet have glucose in his or her urine from a high blood glucose several hours previously.

There are several brands:

- Diastix
- Clinistix (these only give a semiquantitive result)
- Diabur-Test 5000
- Medi-Test Glucose.

All involve wetting a small patch of reagent adhered to a plastic strip, which the patient passes briefly through the stream of urine or dips into a sample. A change in colour after the recommended period of time (approximately 30 to 60 seconds) denotes the presence of glucose. The amount of colour change can be compared against a quantitative colour chart on the side of the container to estimate the quantity of glucose in the urine. Timing of when the test is performed should be varied and the results recorded and discussed with the patient's diabetes team. Consistent negative urine test results that are not confirmed with a normal glycosylated haemoglobin (HbA1c) would suggest that the patient's renal threshold for glucose is above normal and, therefore, urine testing is of no value.

Urine testing is not suitable for patients using insulin or people with poor eyesight.

Blood glucose monitoring

At the time of writing, there were 32 different blood glucose meters available, using 21 blood testing strips made by 10 manufacturers. The meters are not available on prescription but can be purchased quite cheaply from pharmacists, or may be given free of charge by the patient's diabetes or practice nurse (who usually receives them free of charge from the meter manufacturers) (Fig. 4.1). Each meter requires a specific blood glucose-monitoring strip, which is available on prescription (but costs the NHS approximately £14 to £16 for 50 tests). The meters generally feature a simple technique, give a result within a minute or less and require a very small sample of blood. Blood glucose concentrations that can be measured range from 0.6 to 33.3 mmol/l. The meters are designed to give a reasonable measurement of prevailing capillary blood glucose but they are not accurate enough to be used to diagnose diabetes (a venous sample must be used to

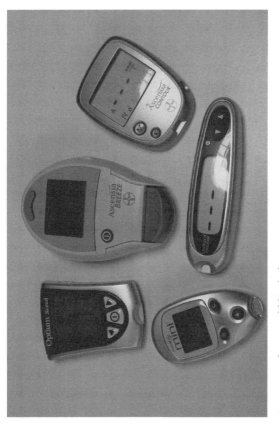

Fig. 4.1 A selection of blood glucose meters.

confirm an abnormal capillary reading; see World Health Organization Guidelines in Table 3.4).

How often to test

There are consensus guidelines now available that recommend frequency of home blood glucose monitoring according to the type of diabetes and treatment (Table 4.1; Owens *et al.*, 2004). However, whether testing is useful and how frequently it should be done should be discussed with the patient as part of their annual diabetes management plan. Patients need to know the range of blood glucose results that they are aiming for, and they should also know what to do if their test results are outside this range on a regular basis.

Patient education

When prescribing test strips, the prescriber should ensure that the patient knows how to calibrate their meter with each new packet of strips, how to use the finger-pricking or lancing device (Fig. 4.2) correctly, the importance of hand-washing before the procedure, how to get an adequate sample of blood (Fig. 4.3), and the correct storage of strips. (They should be stored at room temperature, not in the fridge.)

Pricking their fingers is painful for most patients. Using a new lancet for each test and pricking the side of the finger will make the procedure less uncomfortable. Avoiding the thumb and forefinger may be helpful (these digits are

Table 4.1 Recommendations regarding frequency of blood glucose self-monitoring

Type of diabetes	Monitoring regimen
Type 1	Should consider testing four or more times per day
Diabetes and pregnancy	At least four times per day, especially if using insulin. In patients treated with insulin, testing may need to be more frequent in the first trimester as risk of hypoglycaemia is higher during this time
Type 2 diabetes on basal bolus regimen	At least four times per day
Type 2 diabetes using twice daily insulin and stable glucose control	Test two or three times per week
Type 2 diabetes using twice daily insulin but not stable glucose control	Test at least once daily at varying times
Type 2 diabetes on daily insulin	Test once daily, initially before breakfast until in target range, then daily at varying times
Type 2 diabetes on diet and exercise	Not required
Type 2 diabetes taking metformin or/and glitazone alone	Not required
Type 2 diabetes taking suphonylureas	May be useful to confirm hypoglycaemia

From Owens *et al.*, 2004.

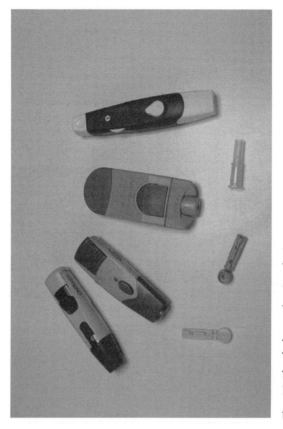

Fig. 4.2 Blood glucose lancing devices.

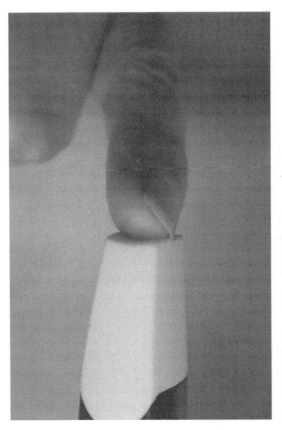

Fig. 4.3 Obtaining a capillary blood glucose sample.

used most frequently in daily life and also skin tends to be thicker). Some meters and lancing devices (e.g. One Touch meters) can be used on alternative sites (e.g. the base of the thumb). The ends of the fingers have a dense network of nerve endings and so are very sensitive. Alternative sites are less painful as they have fewer nerve endings.

The safe disposal of sharps should also be discussed. Sharps should not be thrown away unprotected in household rubbish. Although sharps bins can be prescribed, there should be arrangements in place for the collection and disposal of full bins. This will depend on the local policy in each area.

Testing for ketones

Ketones are produced in significant amounts in conditions of severe insulin deficiency. They result from the metabolism of fats as an alternative energy source when insulin is not available to metabolise glucose in the normal way. Patients with type 1 diabetes are prone to produce ketones if they have missed their insulin injection, injected insufficient amounts of insulin, or their insulin levels are inadequate for their needs, such as during periods of illness. The production of ketones in significant amounts leads to **diabetic ketoacidosis**, which is a medical emergency (Table 4.2). Testing for ketones during periods of illness or episodes of hyperglycaemia can inform patients with type 1 diabetes about making adjustments to their insulin dose

Table 4.2 Interpreting blood ketone levels

State	Blood concentration (mmol/l)
Normal	< 0.6
Hyperketonaemia	> 1.0
Risk of developing diabetic ketoacidosis	> 1.5
Ketoacidosis	> 3.0

or giving extra doses to prevent the development of significant ketosis. Patients with type 1 diabetes should be prescribed ketone-testing equipment for use in these situations. They should be advised to be aware of the expiry date of their strips, however, as they may be out of date if there is no occasion to use them for a long time.

Signs and symptoms of diabetic ketoacidosis are:

- osmotic symptoms
- high blood glucose readings
- dehydration
- anorexia
- drowsiness
- abdominal pain
- nausea and vomiting
- fruity odour ('pear drops') on breath.

As patients with type 2 diabetes still produce insulin, they rarely develop ketones even with marked hyperglycaemia (insulin suppresses the formation of ketones) so the routine prescribing of ketone-testing equipment is not necessary.

However, when assessing any patient with either type 1 or type 2 diabetes who presents as unwell with hyperglycaemia, and particularly vomiting and abdominal pain, a test for either urine or blood ketones is essential.

Testing strips are available for assessing ketones in urine or blood. The Optium Xceed meters can test for both blood glucose and blood ketones simply by changing the testing strip (Abbott Diabetes 01628 678900). Urine testing strips are also available:

- Ketostix
- Ketur test.

These strips are dipped briefly into a urine sample and the change in colour after the prescribed period of time correlates with the amount of ketones in the urine. However, ketones may persist in the urine for several hours after they have disappeared from the blood, so urine testing should be used in conjunction with frequent blood glucose testing and assessment of well-being. Faster clearance of ketones from the blood means blood ketone strips can give a more accurate assessment of possible ketosis (American Diabetes Association, 2004).

REFERENCES

American Diabetes Association (2004) Tests of glycaemia in diabetes. *Diabetes Care* **27**(Suppl. 1): S91–3.

Diabetes Control and Complications Trial Research Group (1993) The effect of intensive treatment of diabetes on the development and progression of long-term complications in insulin-dependent diabetes mellitus. *New England Journal of Medicine* **329**: 977–86.

DoH (2001) *National Service Framework for Diabetes: Standards.* London: The Stationery Office.

Diabetes Prevention Program Research Group (2002) The diabetes prevention program: reduction in the incidence of type 2 diabetes with lifestyle intervention or metformin. *New England Journal of Medicine* **340**: 343–403.

Franciosi M., Pellegrini F., De Beradis G. *et al.* (2001) The impact of blood glucose self-monitoring on metabolic control and quality of life in type 2 diabetic patients: an urgent need for better educational strategies. *Diabetes Care* **24**: 1870–7.

Haffner S. M., Lehto S., Ronnemaa T. *et al.* (1998) Mortality from coronary heart disease in subjects with type 2 diabetes and in nondiabetic subjects with and without prior myocardial infarction. *New England Journal of Medicine* **339**(4): 229–34.

Owens D., Barnett A. H., Kerr D. *et al.* (2004) Blood glucose self-monitoring in type 1 and type 2 diabetes: reaching a multidisciplinary consensus. *Diabetes and Primary Care* **6**: 8–16.

UK Prospective Diabetes Study (UKPDS) Group (1998) Intensive blood-glucose control with sulphonylureas or insulin compared with conventional treatment and risk of complications in patients with type 2 diabetes (UKPDS 33). *Lancet* **352**: 837–53.

RELEVANT NICE GUIDELINES

Orlistat for obesity in adults. *Technology Appraisal* No. 22, March 2001.

Sibutramine for obesity in adults. *Technology Appraisal* No. 31, October 2001.

Guidance on the use of surgery to aid weight reduction for people with morbid obesity. *Technical Appraisal Guidance* No. 46, July 2002.

Management of type 2 diabetes: management of blood glucose. *Inherited Clinical Guideline G*, September 2002.

Guidance on the use of patient-education models in diabetes. *Technology Appraisal* No. 60, 2003.

Brief interventions and referral for smoking cessation in primary care and other settings. *Public Health Intervention Guidance* No. 1; *Technology Appraisal* No. 39, March 2006.

Guidance on the prevention, identification, assessment and management of overweight and obesity in adults and children. *Clinical Guideline* 43, December 2006.

Chapter 5

Management of glycaemia by oral hypoglycaemic agents

Type 2 diabetes is characterised by insulin resistance and a progressive decrease in beta cell function over time. This is reflected in the addition of one then two and even three oral hypoglycaemic agents to the lifestyle modifications made by the patient, with eventually most people requiring insulin therapy to supplement their own insulin production. The aim of this stepwise approach to glycaemic management is to achieve and maintain as near normal glucose levels as possible without inducing unacceptable levels of hypoglycaemia (Box 5.1).

The rationale for controlling blood glucose is to alleviate or prevent symptoms (commonly thirst, polyuria and fatigue), which affect the patient's quality of life, and also to reduce the risk of diabetes complications. The UK Prospective Diabetes Study (UKPDS) demonstrated that any decrease in hyperglycaemia will decrease the risk and severity of diabetic complications. For every 1% decrease in HbA1c (a glycosylated haemoglobin) over 10 years, the risk of myocardial infarction is reduced by 14% and that of microvascular complications by approximately 25%.

Most patients should be supported to aim for a target HbA1c of 7% or less, particularly in the presence of

---

Box 5.1 Target for glycaemic control

HbA1c: 6.5–7.5% (ideally 7% or less)
  Capillary blood glucose:

- 4–6 mmol/l fasting
- < 10 mmol/l after meals.

---

diabetes complications. However, for some individuals, there may be a compromise between accepting less than perfect glycaemic control and reducing the risk of hypoglycaemia. This is particularly relevant when supporting frail elderly patients with diabetes, especially if they live alone. It is also important to remember that any reduction in HbA1c will give benefits, even if the ideal target is not achieved (Stratton *et al.*, 2000).

All pharmacological agents for reducing blood glucose should be in addition to following a healthy lifestyle, not instead of! Patients should be encouraged to follow a healthy eating plan, reduce calorie intake if overweight and increase physical activity to 30 minutes on at least five days a week. Depending on the patient's starting point, this may have to be gradually built up over a period of time. Activity that can be incorporated into the daily routine is likely to be more successful, such as walking more briskly, gardening, and walking instead of driving to local destinations. The activity should be at such a level that the patient feels warm and slightly out of breath but still able to talk. When advising patients about increasing

> **Box 5.2 Patients who may not benefit from increasing physical activity**
>
> Comorbidities that may cause problems with physical activity include:
> - acute foot problems such as neuropathic ulcers (weight-bearing exercise)
> - peripheral neuropathy where patients have very poor sensation in their feet (and are unable to detect blister formation); patients may walk with an abnormal gait, causing callus formation in novel areas of pressure
> - unstable angina or heart disease
> - proliferative retinopathy (avoid exercise that involves straining or lifting).

physical activity, be aware of possible areas of caution or contraindication. Physical activity may not be suitable for some patients (Box 5.2).

Most practitioners will encourage patients with newly diagnosed type 2 diabetes to try and control blood glucose levels initially by following a healthy lifestyle, as recommended by NICE guidelines for type 2 diabetes (Box 5.3). Increasing physical activity and losing weight improves insulin sensitivity and may enable beta cell production of sufficient insulin to meet the needs of reduced insulin resistance and normalise blood glucose levels. However, many patients with type 2 diabetes have had the condition for a number of years before diagnosis,

Box 5.3 Healthy eating advice for all patients with diabetes

- Eat regular meals.
- '5 a day' (of fruit and vegetables).
- Each meal should contain complex starchy foods. Total carbohydrates should make up 45–60% of intake.
- Monounsaturated fat and total carbohydrate should provide 60–70% of energy intake.
- Avoid obvious sugars (e.g. use artificial sweeteners instead of sugar, use diet fizzy drinks) but it is not necessary to exclude all sugar from the diet.
- Fats should not exceed 30% of total calorie intake. Saturated fats should be reduced (e.g. cut the fat off meat before cooking, use a skimmed or semi-skimmed milk), and monounsaturated fats are preferable to polyunsaturated fats (e.g. olive-based spreads are preferable to butter or polyunsaturated spreads, olive oil and pure vegetable and rapeseed oil is better than sunflower oil).
- Eat one or two portions of oily fish per week.
- Total daily salt intake should not exceed 6 g sodium chloride.

From the Nutrition Committee of the Diabetes Care Advisory Committee of Diabetes UK (2003).

and increasing glucose intolerance for a long time before that, so diabetes complications may already be present in these patients. The introduction of metformin at diagnosis, in conjunction with lifestyle advice, has, therefore, been recently recommended by a consensus guideline by the American Diabetes Association and the European Association for the Study of Diabetes for this reason (Nathan *et al.*, 2006). However, it must be emphasised that no matter which oral hypoglycaemic agent (or insulin) is prescribed, it is unlikely to normalise glucose levels if the patient's diet and lifestyle are poor.

Assessment

A patient history should include questioning about signs and symptoms of hyperglycaemia:

- thirst, dry mouth
- polyuria, nocturia (and what volume of urine is passed: if the patient complains of frequency of small amounts of urine, particularly if associated with pain or discomfort, then this is more likely to be caused by a urinary tract infection)
- fatigue (patients often describe feeling tired even when they wake up in the morning or falling asleep when watching the television)
- changes in weight (unintentional weight loss can be a sign of beta cell failure)

- mood changes: irritability, feeling depressed, tearful
- blurred vision or visual changes (patient may describe visiting the optician frequently because their spectacles are not right)
- recurrent vaginal thrush in women and balanitis in men
- in patients with established type 2 diabetes who are self-monitoring, their blood glucose readings are higher than their agreed target range (> 6 mmol/l before breakfast, $\geq$ 10 mmol/l after meals)
- the HbA1c of patients with suboptimal glycaemic control will be higher than 7%.

Possible causes should be checked:

- not adhering to a healthy eating plan (for example, over the Christmas period)
- less physical activity than usual
- recent or current infection (e.g. influenza, urinary tract infection)
- introduction of steroids (e.g. for acute exacerbation of asthma).

Which oral hypoglycaemic agent?

Patients should be treated intensively to achieve their target HbA1c within six months of diagnosis, so if lifestyle alone is not achieving this, pharmacological agents should be added at an early stage and titrated every few weeks to reach the effective dose. Unfortunately, many patients have years of suboptimal glycaemic control because agents are not added or titrated sufficiently quickly.

There are several classes of oral hypoglycaemic agent, with new agents in development. They can be broadly divided into those agents that address the underlying insulin resistance found in most people with type 2 diabetes by improving insulin sensitivity, and those that stimulate the beta cells to increase insulin production. Patients with insulin resistance have normal weight or are usually overweight; they often describe finding it difficult to lose weight, and they may not notice any symptoms of hyperglycaemia. They have also usually been diagnosed relatively recently. Patients who have had diabetes for a number of years, or who describe unintentional weight loss, and often have osmotic symptoms are more likely to need an agent that stimulates the beta cells to produce more insulin, or insulin therapy. Be aware that rapid weight loss and osmotic symptoms in a patient with newly diagnosed diabetes may be a sign that the patient has type 1 diabetes and needs to start insulin rather than oral therapy.

In general, oral hypoglycaemic agents will lower HbA1c by about 1 to 1.5%, so adding in more of these agents may not be appropriate in patients with an HbA1c of > 9% already on one agent. Certain patients will need referral for specialist care (Box 5.4).

Box 5.4 Patients requiring specialist referral

- Patients who continue to lose weight unintentionally despite improvements in home blood glucose monitoring results and HbA1c (for exclusion of other morbidity)
- Patients requiring insulin therapy (unless the practitioner is trained to do this)
- Patients with rapidly deteriorating renal function (> 5 ml/min per year) or those with a glomerular filtration rate < 30 ml/min per 1.73 m^3
- Patients with newly diagnosed type 1 diabetes
- Patients with diabetic ketoacidosis (DKA) or hyperosmolar non-ketotic coma (HONK)
- Patients with poorly controlled diabetes and infection (e.g. infected foot ulcer)
- Women with type 2 diabetes taking oral hypoglycaemic therapy who are planning a pregnancy.

Agents for lowering insulin resistance

There are two classes of oral agent that address insulin resistance: **biguanides** (only metformin now prescribed) and **glitazones**. Apart from improving blood glucose levels by helping the patient to use their own endogenous insulin more effectively, there is evidence that they may have benefits in reducing cardiovascular risk. Information from trials of the glitazones also shows that addressing insulin resistance may slow the progression of type 2 diabetes and delay the necessity for insulin.

Metformin

The first oral hypoglycaemic agent to be introduced for most patients with type 2 diabetes who are not achieving glycaemic control with lifestyle improvements, especially for those who are overweight, is metformin. This is the only remaining example of the biguanide class. This drug is cheap and has been available for a long time. It has enjoyed a renaissance following the UK Prospective Diabetes Study Group (1998) report (UKPDS 34), where metformin not only improved glycaemic control but also reduced mortality in overweight people. However, it commonly causes gastrointestinal side-effects (anorexia, nausea, diarrhoea) and about 10–20% of patients are unable to tolerate the drug. These effects are reduced if the tablet is taken with or after food, and the dose is increased gradually (at two week intervals) starting with 500 mg daily building up to 1 g twice daily (with breakfast and evening meals). If a dose of higher than 2 g is required, this may be best given as a 850 mg tablet three times a day, with meals. A slow-release form (Glucophage SR) may be better tolerated in those patients who cannot tolerate the usual formulation (and it has the advantage that the full dose, 2 g, can all be given at one time with the evening meal, which may help in compliance).

Metformin is usually maintained when patients change to insulin, as it reduces the amount of injected insulin required and may limit the weight gain often seen in patients starting insulin.

Mode of action. The exact action of metformin is unclear but it appears to reduce hepatic glucose production, decrease intestinal absorption of glucose and improve insulin sensitivity (by increasing peripheral glucose uptake and utilisation). It does not stimulate the beta cells and, therefore, does not cause hypoglycaemia or weight gain when used as monotherapy.

Contraindications. It should not be used in patients with conditions that predispose to lactic acidosis such as renal impairment (serum creatinine of > 140 mmol/l in women, 150 mmol/l in men, or an estimated glomerular filtration rate of ≤ 30 ml/min per 1.72 m^3), hepatic impairment, recent myocardial infarction, heart failure, respiratory failure, shock or trauma, or those with a high alcohol intake.

Caution. As diarrhoea is a relatively common side-effect, metformin should be used with caution in patients who already are prone to this (e.g. Chrohn's disease, irritable bowel syndrome). It should be temporarily discontinued (for 48 hours) in patients undergoing radiological investigations involving the use of intravenous iodinated contrast such as an intravenous pyelogram and for any surgical procedures until normal food intake is resumed.

Side-effects.   Lactic acidosis can rarely (less than 1% of patients) occur as result of metformin accumulation, especially in patients with renal failure. Metformin commonly (in more than 10% of patients) causes gastrointestinal side-effects including nausea, vomiting, diarrhoea and flatulence. Less commonly, it may cause indigestion and a metallic taste in the mouth. It may also decrease the absorption of vitamin B_{12} and folic acid.

Monitoring.   Serum creatinine should be measured at least annually (metformin is excreted by the kidneys) and signs and symptoms of vitamin B_{12} and/or folic acid deficiency should be checked. Glycated haemoglobin (HbA1c), at least annually, is used to check efficacy in maintaining normoglycaemia.

Glitazones

If the patient is of normal weight or overweight and still not achieving glycaemic control, the next drug of choice is usually a glitazone. NICE (2002) recommends that for people with type 2 diabetes, glitazone should only be used as second-line therapy added to either metformin or a sulphonylurea, as an alternative to a combination of metformin and a sulphonylurea in those who are unable to take this combination because of intolerance or contraindication to one of the drugs. However, increased use of glitazones in the management of insulin resistance has led the Association of British Consultant Diabetologists to issue a consensus statement that encourages such use as an alternative to sulphonylureas in these patients (Higgs and Krentz, 2004). The glitazones are licensed for use as monotherapy, dual and triple therapy. Pioglitazone (Actos) and Rosiglitazone (Avandia) are the two drugs available in this class. The first glitazone, troglitazone, was swiftly removed soon after launch as it was found to cause fatal liver disease in a small number of patients.

This class of drug (also known as the thiazolidinediones or PPAR-gamma agonists) has no direct effect on insulin production (therefore will not cause hypoglycaemia as monotherapy or with metformin) but tackles insulin resistance by improving insulin sensitivity, particularly in adipose tissue, and reducing glucose production by the liver.

Patients need to be warned that glitazones take at least six weeks to show any improvement in blood glucose, and, therefore, they would not be the drug of choice if the patient has significant hyperglycaemia symptoms as they take so long to have an effect.

Both glitazones increase the risk of heart failure. They can cause fluid retention and are therefore *absolutely* contraindicated in patients with a history of heart failure. At the time of publication of this book, there has been considerable debate about the safety of glitazones, following the publication of a meta-analysis of studies involving rosiglitazone (Nissan and Wolski, 2007), which showed that there was an increased risk of myocardial infarction in patients using this drug. The cardiovascular benefit of the other glitazone, pioglitazone, was investigated in the PROactive Study (Dormandy *et al.*, 2005). Although the study, which involved patients with type 2 diabetes and established cardiovascular disease, failed to meet its primary endpoint, which was a composite of death, myocardial infarction, acute coronary syndrome, stroke and various surgical procedures, it did show a reduction in risk of recurrent myocardial infarction and stroke in these high-risk patients.

An interesting side-effect was noted in the ADOPT trial recently (Khan *et al.*, 2006), which suggested that there was a significantly increased risk of fractures in women who were taking rosiglitazone compared with metformin or sulphonylureas. The fractures occurred in the wrist, humerus and foot, not areas associated with postmenopausal osteoporosis, and the underlying cause has not been determined. A similar effect has also been found in women taking pioglitazone (Schwarz and Sellmeyer, 2007). This should be taken into account when considering using a glitazone in women, particularly those with a history of bone problems or falls.

Patients who take both metformin and a glitazone may prefer a combined formulation: Avandamet, which is metformin and rosiglitazone, or the recently licensed Competact (metformin and pioglitazone).

Mode of action. Glitazones mainly act on a nuclear receptor PPAR-gamma, which is most strongly expressed in adipose tissue. The receptor increases the transcription of certain insulin-sensitive genes involved in the metabolism of lipids and glucose, thereby lowering insulin resistance.

Contraindications. Glitazones should not be used in patients with a history of cardiac failure or liver impairment. Until recently, they were contraindicated for use with insulin as initially there was evidence that this could increase the risk of heart failure. However, the two agents have been used together with insulin for years in the USA without significant problems, so this contraindication has been withdrawn. Pioglitazone, however, is the only formulation to have a licence for use with insulin.

Cautions. Glitazones should be stopped 48 hours before surgery and not restarted for 48 hours afterwards. They should also be stopped for 48 hours after tests using iodinated contrast agents. As glitazones improve insulin sensitivity, ovulation can resume in women with polycystic ovary syndrome or those who are anovulatory because of insulin resistance. Glitazones are eliminated by the CYP2C8 system and so require caution if used with CYP2C8 inhibitors (e.g. gemfibrozil) or inducers (e. g. rifampicin). Following recent evidence of increased risk of fractures in women using glitazones, this should be considered when prescribing them for women with any condition that already increases the risk of fractures (e.g. those with a history of falls).

Side-effects. Fluid retention can exacerbate or precipitate heart failure. Peripheral oedema may cause swelling of the ankles. It can also cause a reduced haematocrit and decrease in haemoglobin, leading to anaemia if haemoglobin levels are low when glitazones are initiated. Weight gain is also a problem.

Monitoring. The first glitazone, troglitazone, had to be withdrawn because of several cases of fatal liver toxicity. Although the two glitazones currently in use show no evidence of causing liver problems, liver function tests were recommended when they were first introduced. It is still usual practice to check liver function occasionally (e.g. as part of the diabetes annual review). Patients should be monitored for weight gain, and questioned about ankle oedema and symptoms of anaemia.

Dosage. The following tablets are available:
– Rosiglitazone: 4 or 8 mg
– Pioglitazone: 15, 30 or 45 mg
– Avandamet (rosiglitazone plus metformin): 2/500, 2/1000 or 4/1000 mg
– Competact (pioglitazone plus metformin): 15/850 mg.

Agents that stimulate beta cells to produce more insulin

Sulphonylureas

Sulphonylureas stimulate the beta cells to release more insulin (and, therefore, are dependent on the patient having some residual beta cell function). In the individual

> **Box 5.5 Signs and symptoms of hypoglycaemia (see Chapter 7)**
>
> All patients taking sulphonylureas, prandial regulators and insulin therapy should be aware of the signs and symptoms of hypoglycaemia: sudden onset of sweating, trembling, headache, hunger, 'jitteriness', feeling faint, anxiety, palpitations, confusion and coma. They should be advised to carry glucose with them at all times.

without diabetes, insulin production by the beta cells is reduced as blood sugar reaches the lower end of the normal glucose range. As sulphonylureas override this feedback system, these drugs can cause hypoglycaemia. As sulphonylureas are excreted by the kidney, patients with any degree of renal impairment are at increased risk of hypoglycaemic episodes (Box 5.5). Weight gain is another unwanted effect of this class of drug.

Sulphonylureas work quickly and will allieviate hyperglycaemic symptoms within a few days. They are also the first-line choice in patients who are thin and already following a healthy diet, but these patients require frequent monitoring as they may have type 1 diabetes, and, therefore, require insulin.

There are five agents in this class, varying in duration of action:

- tolbutamide: oldest example; 500 mg three times a day before meals

- glibenclamide: 2.5 to 15 mg daily; action may last more than 24 hours and so is not recommended for the elderly
- gliclazide: 40 mg daily to 160 mg twice a day
- glimeperide: 1 to 6 mg daily
- glipizide: 2.5 to 15 mg daily.

Gliquidone has recently been discontinued.

Gliclazide is the most commonly prescribed sulphonylurea. Gliclazide MR is a slow-release formulation (30 to 120 mg daily) and may reduce risk of hypoglycaemia and, as taken daily, may improve compliance.

Prandial regulators

There are two examples of prandial regulators currently available: repaglinide (formerly marketed as Novonorm but recently renamed Prandin) and nateglinide (Starlix). These drugs are rapid-acting insulin secretagogues: they stimulate the beta cells within approximately 10–30 minutes of ingestion to release a short bolus of insulin that mimics the bolus of insulin produced by the non-diabetic individual after a carbohydrate load. As the class name suggests, they are taken before a meal to reduce the postprandial rise in blood glucose. As they stimulate insulin production, they can cause hypoglycaemia, but as they are short acting (approximately 2–4 hours duration), they are less likely to cause weight gain. They are taken just before a main meal, so are useful for patients who have an erratic meal pattern. If a meal is missed, the tablet should be missed too. (This may be useful for patients who fast, during Ramadan for example.) However, they have little effect on basal insulin levels so may not achieve normal pre-breakfast blood glycaemia as monotherapy. They are usually taken in conjunction with metformin; indeed the Starlix licence is not for monotherapy but in addition to metformin.

They should not be prescribed in addition to sulphonylureas, and the concomitant use of repaglinide and gemfibrozil is contraindicated.

Other hypoglycaemic agents

Alpha-glucosidase inhibitors

Acarbose (Glucobay) is the only example available in this class. The enzyme glucosidase, which facilitates the breakdown of carbohydrates into monosaccharides for their absorption in the small intestine, is inhibited by acarbose. It has very little effect on fasting blood glucose but can reduce the rise of postprandial blood glucose. It can be used as monotherapy but usually is used in combination with any other oral hypoglycaemic agent or insulin. Unfortunately, the side-effects of flatulence, abdominal pain and diarrhoea often mean the patient cannot tolerate the drug (Holman *et al.*, 1999). As this drug inhibits breakdown of carbohydrate into glucose, patients who are at risk of hypoglycaemia should be advised to use only glucose to treat hypoglycaemic episodes, not starchy foods.

Incretin mimics

The incretins are hormones produced by the L cells in the wall of the small intestine in response to a carbohydrate meal. They have a number of effects including stimulating the short burst of insulin release associated with eating. In people with type 2 diabetes, the incretin effect is impaired, and loss of mealtime insulin response is one of the early signs of impaired glucose tolerance. Glucagon-like peptide 1 (GLP-1) is an incretin for which an artificial analogue has been developed. This agent, exenatide (Byetta) needs to be injected twice daily, up to 60 minutes before breakfast and the evening meal. It is currently licensed for use with metformin or sulphonylureas or a combination of both. The agent is introduced at 5 μg (micrograms) twice daily for the first month and then changed to 10 μg twice daily if tolerated. Oral GLP-1 agents are being developed.

Exenatide is available in 5 and 10 μg disposable Byetta pens (Fig. 5.1), for which insulin pen needles are required. Suitable injection sites, technique and disposal of sharps are as recommended for insulin injections (see Chapter 6).

Although exenatide is given by an injection, it does not have the same HGV and PSV driving licence restriction that insulin has, so it may be a useful treatment choice for someone who is resisting insulin therapy for this reason. However, as the agent improves beta cell insulin production, it relies on a reasonable beta cell mass still being available. Someone who has had diabetes for many

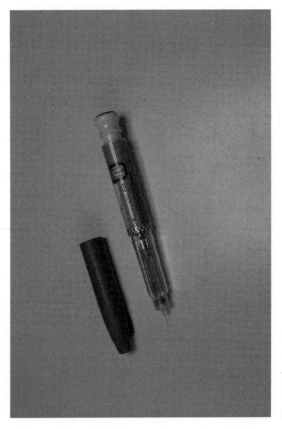

Fig. 5.1 The Byetta pen.

years, particularly if they have unintentional weight loss, is less likely to respond to exenatide as their functioning beta cell mass will be insufficient.

Mode of action. In response to a carbohydrate meal, GLP-1 stimulates a glucose-dependent insulin secretion from the beta cells. This means that it is unlikely to cause hypoglycaemia unless used with a sulphonylurea. It suppresses glucagon secretion from the alpha cells in the pancreas, which suppresses hepatic glucose output. It has effects in the central nervous system that promote satiety and reduce appetite; it also delays gastric emptying, which further reduces appetite. The latter two actions promote weight loss.

Contraindications. Pancreatitis is a potential side-effect, so exenatide should be avoided in those at risk of this (e.g. with high alcohol intake). It is not suitable for patients who have type 1 diabetes or patients with type 2 and significant beta cell failure.

Caution. As exenatide stimulates insulin production and reduces appetite, the risk of hypoglycaemia is increased with patients also using sulphonylureas. If HbA1c is $< 8\%$, it is advisable to reduce these agents and monitor blood glucose levels. The sulphonylureas can be slowly increased again if blood glucose levels are suboptimal and there is no evidence of hypoglycaemia. Patients using the oral contraceptive pill, proton pump inhibitors or antibiotics should be advised to take these about an hour before meals.

Side-effects.   Nausea, vomiting and diarrhoea are
very common. Hypoglycaemia may occur if the
patient is also using sulphonylureas. A small
number of cases of pancreatitis have been
reported; these usually resolved if exenatide was
discontinued.

Monitoring.   There is no need for additional home
blood glucose monitoring unless it is used in
conjunction with sulphonylureas. Once the patient is
established on exenatide, this additional monitoring
can be discontinued.

Dipeptidyl peptidase 4 inhibitors

The incretins are rapidly inactivated by the enzyme
dipeptidyl peptidase 4 (DPP-4). The first agent to
inhibit DPP-4, sitagliptin (Januvia), became available
in May 2007, with vildagliptin (Galvus) due in 2008
and others to follow. These agents prolong the
availability of naturally occurring incretin. Sitagliptin is
taken orally, once a day and appears to have a very low
side-effect profile. It is licenced for use in patients with
type 2 diabetes in combination with metformin or a
glitazone, and ideally it should be used in the early
stages of diabetes. As it is weight neutral, it is an
attractive option for patients who need to reduce their
HbA1c but who are overweight.

Table 5.1 summarises the main non-insulin agents for
blood glucose control.

Table 5.1 Summary of the main non-insulin agents available for lowering glucose

Name	Dose	Action	Main side-effects
Biguanide			
Metformin (Glucophage, Glucophage MR)	Start with 500 mg and increase usually to 1 g bd with food over several weeks	Decreases production of glucose by the liver; improves glucose uptake by skeletal muscles	Gastrointestinal: nausea, anorexia, diarrhoea, metallic taste in mouth
Glitazones			
Rosiglitazone (Avandia)	4–8 mg daily	Improve insulin sensitivity and reduce insulin resistance	Fluid retention, heart failure, weight gain; may increase risk of fractures in women
Pioglitazone (Actos)	15–45 mg daily		
Sulphonylureas			
Gliclazide	40 mg daily up to 160 mg bd	Stimulate beta cells to produce more insulin	Hypoglycaemia; weight gain
Gliclazide MR	30–120 mg daily		
Glipizide	2.5–15 mg daily, up to 20 mg if dose divided		

Table 5.1 (*cont.*)

Name	Dose	Action	Main side-effects
Glibenclamide	2.5–15 mg daily		
Glimepiride	1–6 mg daily		
Tolbutamide	500 mg daily up to tds		
Prandial regulators			
Repaglinide, (Prandin formerly Novonorm)	0.5–4 mg with meals up to maximum of 16 mg per day	Stimulate beta cells to produce short-lasting mealtime bolus of insulin	Hypoglycaemia
Nataglinide (Starlix)	60–180 mg tds (licensed with metformin, not monotherapy)		
Alpha-glucosidase inhibitor			
Acarbose (Glucobay)	50–200 mg tds; take with first mouthful of meal	Reduces carbohydrate absorption from the gut	Gastrointestinal: flatulence, diarrhoea, bloating, abdominal pain
Incretin mimic			
Exenatide (Byetta)	5 micrograms bd for first month	Stimulates beta cells in response to	Nausea, vomiting and diarrhoea

Name	Dose	Action	Main side-effects
	then 10 micrograms bd injections	carbohydrate; reduces hepatic glucose output; slows down gastric emptying and promotes satiety	
Dipeptidyl peptidase 4 inhibitor			
Sitagliptin (Januvia)	100 mg daily	Stimulates carbohydrate-related insulin production by the beta cell	Generally well tolerated

bd, twice daily; tds, three times a day.

Which oral hypoglycaemic agent?

A number of factors must be taken into consideration when deciding which oral hypoglycaemic agent to prescibe. The two case studies below feature women with many similarities but needing a different regimen.

Jennifer, aged 41 years, type 2 diabetes, BMI 31, HbA1c 8%, currently taking metformin 1 g twice a day

Always reinforce lifestyle advice

Options:

- consider anti-obesity medication to reduce weight and, therefore, insulin resistance
- add in a glitazone to tackle insulin resistance (but this may cause weight gain, fluid retention and increase risk of fractures)
- add in a DPP4 inhibitor, which is weight neutral (but limited clinical experience available)
- add in twice daily injections of exenatide (this may help her to lose weight as well as reduce her HbA1c, but can cause nausea)
- add in a sulphonylurea (but this may increase weight and cause hypoglycaemia)
- add in insulin (but this may increase weight and risk of hypoglycaemia).

Susan aged 41 years, type 2 diabetes, BMI 31, HbA1c 9.5%, currently on metformin 1 g twice a day

Although Susan appears similar to Jennifer, her option for the addition of another oral hypoglycaemic agent may be limited as these are unlikely to reduce her HbA1c by more than 1% and she will not achieve her target of 7% or less; consequently, the addition of insulin may be more appropriate.

REFERENCES

Dormandy J. A., Charbonnel B., Eckland D. J. A. *et al.* (2005) Secondary prevention of macrovascular events in patients with type 2 diabetes in the PROactive Study (PROspective pioglitAzone Clinical Trial In macroVascular Events): a randomised controlled trial. *Lancet* **366**: 1279–89.

Higgs E. R., and Krentz A. J. (2004) Association of British Clinical Diabetologists position statement on glitazones. *Practical Diabetes International* **21**: 1–3.

Holman R. R., Cull C. A. and Turner R. C. (1999) A randomized double-blind trial of acarbose in type 2 diabetes shows improved glycemic control over 3 years (UK Prospective Diabetes Study 44). *Diabetes Care* **22**: 960–4.

Khan S. E., Haffner S. M., Heise M. A. *et al.* (2006) Glycaemic durability of rosiglitazone, metformin or glyburide monotherapy. *New England Journal of Medicine* **355**: 2427–43.

Nathan D. M., Buse J. B., Davidson M. B. *et al.* (2006) Management of hyperglycaemia in type 2 diabetes: a consensus algorithm for the initiation and adjustment of therapy. *Diabetologia* **49**: 1711–21.

Nissan S. E., and Wolski K. (2007) Effect of rosiglitazone on the risk of myocardial infarction and death from cardiovascular causes. *New England Journal of Medicine* **356**: 2457–71.

Nutrition Committee of the Diabetes Care Advisory Committee of Diabetes UK (2003) The implementation of nutritional advice for people with diabetes. *Diabetic Medicine* **20**: 786–807.

Schwartz A. V., and Sellmeyer D. E. (2007) Thiazolidinedione therapy gets complicated. Is bone loss the price of improved insulin resistance? *Diabetes Care* **30**: 1670–71.

Stratton I. M., Adler A. I., Neil H. A. *et al.* (2000) Association of glycaemia with macrovascular and microvascular complications of type 2 diabetes (UKPDS 35): prospective observational study. *British Medical Journal* **321**: 405–12.

UK Prospective Diabetes Study (UKPDS) Group (1998) Effect of intensive blood-glucose control with metformin on complications in overweight patients with diabetes (UKPDS 34). *Lancet* **352**: 854–65.

RELEVANT NICE GUIDELINES

Management of type 2 diabetes: management of blood glucose. *Inherited Clinical Guideline G*, September 2002.

Diabetes (type 2): glitazones *Technology Appraisal* No. 63, August 2003.

Management of type 2 diabetes is currently being updated and will be published in summer 2008.

Chapter 6

Insulin therapy

Insulin production in the person without diabetes can be described as having two components. A constant 'background' or basal production maintains fasting blood glucose between 3.5 and 6 mmol/l by controlling glucose production from the liver. A short-acting, rapidly produced 'spike' or bolus of insulin is produced after a carbohydrate meal (see Fig. 3.1). The size of this bolus varies with the size and type of carbohydrate (e.g. a glass of non-diet cola will produce a rapid, high spike whereas a slice of bread would produce a shorter more prolonged spike as this is absorbed over a longer period of time).

The aim of insulin therapy is to achieve near-normal glycaemia without causing hypoglycaemia or unacceptable weight gain. All patients with type 1 diabetes and eventually most people with type 2 diabetes will require insulin therapy. There are a bewildering number of insulins and devices available. The different types of insulin try to mimic either the background (long-acting or intermediate forms) or the mealtime (rapid or short-acting form) insulin, or are a mixture of the two. Which insulins are used will depend on the relative insulin deficiency, manual dexterity, visual capacity, age and lifestyle of each patient.

> ### Box 6.1 Target for glycaemic control
>
> HbA1c: 6.5– 7.5%
>
> Capillary blood glucose:
>
> - 4–6 mmol/l fasting
> - < 10 mmol/l after meals.

Types of insulin

Most patients today use human-identical insulins.
These insulins are manufactured using either yeast or
bacteria that have had their DNA altered so they produce
a string of amino acids that are identical to the amino
acid chains that make up the insulin produced by the
non-diabetic individual. The **analogue insulins** are made
from human-identical insulin in which slight changes
have been made in the order or content of the amino acid
chain that gives the insulin additional properties (a longer
smoother profile in the case of the basal analogue insulins
and a rapid short action in the case of the rapid-acting
analogue insulins).

When insulin was first used therapeutically, only
pork or beef insulin derived directly from animals
was available. Some patients are still using these
insulins today (and have survived 30 or more years so
should be allowed to continue on these if that is their
choice) and some patients choose to change to animal
insulins from the modern insulins. There is evidence

Table 6.1 Animal insulins still available

Insulin type	Product
Short-acting mealtime insulin	Hypurin Porcine Neutral
	Hypurin Beef Neutral
Intermediate background insulin	Hypurin Porcine Isophane
	Hypurin Beef Isophane
Insulin mixtures	Hypurin Porcine 30/70 Mix
	Hypurin Beef 30/70 Mix

that some people do not feel well when using modern insulins, with a range of symptoms that may be quite non-specific but affect their general well-being. The Insulin Dependent Diabetes Trust is a patient support group that has promoted the continued availability of animal insulin choice over the years during which all of the three main insulin companies have discontinued their selection of animal insulins. Wockhardt insulins continue to make a limited range of beef-and pork-derived insulins (Table 6.1).

Transferring patients to animal insulins from human-identical insulins is unlikely to cause problems unless the patient has been using analogue insulins, as animal insulins do not have the additional properties that these insulins possess so patients may find it difficult to keep as tight a control when using animal insulins. However, if they feel better generally, it may be a worthwhile compromise.

However, transferring patients who have been using animal insulins for a number of years to human-identical or analogue insulins needs close supervision and specialist support. As the chain of amino acids is different in pork and especially beef insulins, antibodies are built up over the years that the patient has been injecting this foreign protein into their bodies. The dose of insulin injected will have needed to be increased over the years to compensate for this antibody action. If the same dose of human-identical insulin is injected, the patient will have an overdose as antibodies to animal insulin will not recognise this as a foreign protein and the complete dose will have effect. When human-identical insulin was first introduced, there were a number of cases of patients having profound hypoglycaemic episodes until this was recognised. When changing from animal insulin to human identical insulin, therefore, the usual total dose should initially be reduced by about 20% and the patient should monitor their blood glucose frequently until their levels are stable. The other problem when changing insulin sources is that patients notice they have much stronger and earlier warning symptoms of hypoglycaemia with animal insulins. Patients must be warned that their hypoglycaemia symptoms may change and diminish, and that symptoms that in the past occurred when their blood sugar was about 4 mmol/l may, in fact, not occur until their blood sugar is much lower so they should not delay treatment.

Insulins used to mimic the mealtime bolus

In the individual without diabetes, insulin is produced in response to eating a carbohydrate meal. There is a rapid production of insulin by the beta cells, the amount of which is tailored to the amount and type of carbohydrate. A sugary drink would cause a sharp rise in blood glucose whereas a starchy meal would be digested and the glucose released slowly over several hours, so the boluses of insulin produced by the beta cells would differ in amount and length of time produced. Ideally, insulins that aim to mimic these mealtime boluses should be rapid acting and be adjusted to maintain normal blood glucose with the amount of carbohydrate eaten. There are two types of mealtime insulins: the soluble insulins, which have been available for decades, and the newer rapid-acting analogue insulins.

Short-acting soluble insulins

Short-acting insulins should be injected between 20 and 30 minutes before a meal as they take about an hour to start being effective (Table 6.2). They are not particularly short acting as they can last up to 6 or 8 hours so patients may require a small snack between meals to compensate for this extended action and reduce risk of hypoglycaemia before the next meal. They can be adjusted according to the amount of carbohydrate in the meal. Testing 2 hours after the meal and before the next meal gives an indication of how effective the insulin dose was (e.g. tests 2 hours

Table 6.2 Short-acting mealtime insulins

Name of insulin	Manufacturer
Humulin S	Lilly
Actrapid (vial only)	Novo Nordisk
Insuman rapid	Sanofi Aventis
Hypurin porcine neutral	Wockhardt
Hypurin beef neutral	Wockhardt

after breakfast or before lunch give information about the action of the breakfast insulin). Although these soluble insulins have the disadvantages of needing to be injected some time before the meal and require the patient to take snacks, they can be useful for patients who have a normal pre-breakfast fasting blood glucose but whose fasting blood sugars during the day and pre-bed are above normal despite optimising the basal insulin. The extended action of these insulins, therefore, also provides some basal cover as well as preventing postprandial hyperglycaemia.

Rapid-acting analogue insulins

The limitations of the soluble insulins led to the development of the rapid-acting analogue insulins, of which there are now three (Table 6.3). These produce a rapid sharp rise in insulin, can be given immediately before or after a meal and are effective for approximately 2 to 3 hours. When the dose is manipulated according to the carbohydrate portion of the meal, they can mimic very

Table 6.3 Rapid-acting, meal-time bolus insulins

Name of insulin	Manufacturer
Humalog (Lispro)	Lilly
Novorapid (Aspart)	Novo Nordisk
Glulisine (Apidra)	Sanofi Aventis

closely the mealtime boluses of insulin produced in the non-diabetic individual.

Insulins used to mimic the background (basal) insulins

Until recently, the rapid-acting insulins could replace the mealtime boluses very effectively in people with type 1 diabetes, but the background insulins available did not provide the ideal basal background found in the individual without diabetes. There are now two long-acting basal analogue insulins available that produce a long-acting (24 hours in most patients) relatively smooth profile, which should enable most patients to maintain a normal fasting blood glucose while minimising the risk of hypoglycaemia (Table 6.4). Although these have advantages over the older basal insulins, they are still not perfect, especially if the patient has quite marked differences in basal requirements over 24 hours. These insulins are designed to be released slowly and evenly over time, but a flat profile may not be an advantage in some circumstances. For example, they

Table 6.4 Long-acting, basal/
background insulins

Name of insulin	Manufacturer
Glargine (Lantus)	Sanofi Aventis
Detemir (Levemir)	Novo Nordisk

may cause hypoglycaemia during periods of exercise
(when the basal insulin would be reduced in someone
without diabetes), or they may cause hyperglycaemia
during periods of illness (when the basal requirements
increase owing to the insulin resistance that occurs in
illness). Some patients with type 1 diabetes have marked
'dawn phenomenon', where the early morning growth
hormone surge that occurs normally as part of waking up
causes pronounced insulin resistance. The patient wakes
up with persistently high fasting blood sugars, but if they
try to compensate for this by increasing their basal insulin,
they start to get regular episodes of hypoglycaemia during
the day or early night time. These patients may benefit
from an insulin pump in which the basal component of
their insulin can be programmed to vary hour by hour.

Blood glucose tests before meals, but in particular before
breakfast, give the best information about the effectiveness
of the basal insulin. The dose is adjusted every few days
until the pre-breakfast tests are usually within the ideal
range (which for most people would be between 4 and
6 mmol/l). As these insulins do not peak, they do not need
to be given in relation to food. They are usually given at

bedtime but can be given at any time in the day so long as it is regularly at that time. This is particularly useful for district nurses giving insulin, when it can be difficult to time the injection to the patient's mealtime. Some patients may require Levemir twice daily but Lantus usually gives sufficient effect for 24 hours.

Intermediate background insulin

Before the development of the long-acting basal analogue insulins, many patients used the intermediate or Neutral Protamine Hagedorn (NPH) insulins to provide a basal insulin supply (Table 6.5). Many patients still use these, and as most of their action lasts approximately 12 to 14 hours, they can be useful for patients who have very different basal requirements during the day from their night time requirements (e.g. they may need a small dose of background insulin if they have a very active job in the day, and a larger dose at night when they are not active). Also, this insulin may be used if the device it is available in is the only device that a patient can use independently (and avoids the need for a district nurse). The InnoLet pen device until recently was only available in Insulatard and Mixtard 30, but it is useful for elderly patients as it looks like an egg timer and it is easy to use for people with poor eyesight and manual dexterity problems. Levemir insulin is now available in this device.

These insulins are cloudy: the insulin is mixed with a substance that delays its action. They require resuspension before every injection so patients need to

Table 6.5 Intermediate (NPH) insulins

Name of insulin	Manufacturer
Insulatard	Novo Nordisk
Humulin I	Lilly
Insuman basal	Sanofi Aventis
Hypurin Porcine Isophane	Wockhardt
Hypurin Beef Isophane	Wockhardt

be advised to shake their insulin pen or rotate the vial of insulin at least 10 times before use. Failure to do this can alter the profile of the insulin, causing erratic blood glucose readings.

When used with mealtime insulins in basal bolus regimens, these insulins should be given at a regular time at bedtime. Testing blood glucose before breakfast will inform the patient whether the dose is correct (high fasting tests means they should increase the dose; low tests can be rectified by reducing the dose). These insulins have a marked peak in their profile, during which the patient is at increased risk of hypoglycaemia. This is a particular problem in the night, and eating a supper of complex carbohydrate is recommended when using this insulin (such as toast or cereal).

Mixtures of insulin

As the name suggests, insulin mixtures are a fixed combination of two insulins: a short- or rapid-acting insulin plus an intermediate-acting background insulin. The proportion of mealtime insulin to background insulin is given by the number in the name (e.g. Novomix 30 is made up of 30% Novorapid and 70% Insulatard). As it is a mixture, it is essential that the insulin is resuspended thoroughly before every injection.

When trying to mimic the normal profile of someone without diabetes, the use of separate basal and mealtime insulins is recommended. However, this requires at least four injections a day, frequent blood glucose monitoring and, ideally, a good understanding of carbohydrates and skills in insulin dose adjustment. Some patients may not be able to manage this or, if they have type 2 diabetes and a regular lifestyle and eating pattern, may not require this degree of intensive insulin therapy. For these patients an insulin mixture will give reasonable glycaemic control. Until recently, most patients in the UK with type 2 diabetes requiring insulin were usually started on a twice-daily mixture of insulin.

Mixtures of rapid-acting bolus and intermediate insulins

Mixtures of rapid-acting and intermediate insulins (Table 6.6) should be given shortly before, or at the end, of breakfast and the evening meal. If the mid-afternoon and pre-evening meal blood glucose tests are above normal, a third injection with lunch may be useful. They can also be used as a daily injection with the evening meal when

Table 6.6 Insulin mixtures using rapid-acting analogues

Name	Manufacturer
Novomix 30	Novo Nordisk
Humalog Mix 25	Lilly
Humalog Mix 50	Lilly

Table 6.7 Insulin mixtures using short-acting insulin

Name	Manufacturer
Mixtard 30	Novo Nordisk
Humulin M3	Lilly
Insuman Comb 15	Sanofi Aventis
Insuman Comb 25	Sanofi Aventis
Insuman Comb 50	Sanofi Aventis
Hypurin Porcine 30/70	Wockhardt

starting insulin therapy if hyperglycaemia in the evening and pre-breakfast is the problem.

Mixtures of short-acting bolus and intermediate insulins

As the mealtime insulin is the older type of soluble insulin, mixtures of a short-acting bolus and an intermediate insulin (Table 6.7) should be given 20 to 30 minutes before breakfast and before the evening meal.

Insulin regimens

One or more insulin types are used in insulin regimens for patients requiring insulin, but which types and which regimen will vary with the individual (Table 6.8). An elderly patient with type 2 diabetes living alone and requiring district nurse support would perhaps manage with a simple daily insulin to keep the patient symptom free and minimise the risk of hypoglycaemia. A person with type 1 diabetes would usually require insulins to replace both basal and mealtime insulins as they do not produce any insulin themselves, and so would need at least four injections a day. Someone with a stable lifestyle and regular mealtimes may manage with twice daily regimens. For some patients, the insulin regimen used may be determined by their choice of insulin device.

Some common insulin regimens are now given and Table 6.9 summarises how to adjust the insulin dose within the various regimens.

Daily basal insulin with or without oral hypoglycaemic agents

Inclusion of a daily basal insulin dose is the simplest regimen to use with patients with type 2 diabetes already taking maximum oral hypoglycaemic agents but who are not achieving an HbA1c of 7% or less. The patient

Table 6.8 Which insulin regimen?

Patient	Insulin requirements
Does the patient have type 1 diabetes?	Patients with type 1 diabetes do not produce any insulin and so will usually require basal and mealtime insulins
Does the patient have varying mealtimes and variable meal sizes?	Using a rapid-acting insulin with meals means the patient can inject whenever they eat, whatever time it is, and can adjust the dose to accommodate the varying size of the meal
Does the patient have poor eyesight or manual dexterity problems?	Demonstrate a variety of insulin pen devices (with magnifiers if appropriate) and find a device that the patient is able to use independently. Choose a regimen using the insulin that is available in this device if possible
Is the patient dependent on others to give the injection?	Keep the number of injections required to a minimum, and if possible, use a basal analogue insulin that can be given at any regular time, not related to meals
Is the patient resistant to adding in mealtime injections but despite having a normal pre-breakfast blood glucose on a basal injection, has high tests in the day?	If the patient has a regular lifestyle, changing to a twice-daily insulin from a daily basal insulin will give some mealtime cover with just two injections a day.
Are the pre-breakfast and day time blood tests normal on a basal insulin, but the glucose is high after the main meal of the day?	The patient can add in one mealtime insulin with the main meal (whether that is at lunchtime or evening time) in addition to their basal insulin dose

Table 6.9 When to adjust insulin dose

Insulin regimen	Useful blood testing time	Adjustment
Daily basal analogue	Daily before breakfast	Increase insulin by 2–4 units every three days until blood glucose is between 4 and 6 mmol/l
Twice daily mixture	Vary test times throughout the day	Increase or decrease morning dose by 10% every few days until tests in the day are in acceptable range; increase or decrease evening dose until tests in the evening, night and pre-breakfast are in acceptable range
Basal bolus/ basal plus	Before breakfast and 2 hours after meals	Increase or decrease basal insulin until pre-breakfast test is usually between 4 and 6 mmol/l. Adjust breakfast dose by small increments every few days until the test 2 hours after breakfast is in target (ideally less than 8 mmol/l)
		Adjust midday meal insulin by small increments until the test 2 hours after lunch is in target
		Adjust evening meal insulin by small increments until the test 2 hours after evening meal is in target

continues with the oral therapy and a small single dose (e.g. 10 units) of insulin is introduced. This can be a basal analogue insulin (Lantus or Detemir) at any time of day, an intermediate insulin at bedtime (Insulatard, Insuman basal or Humulin I) or a rapid-acting mixture with the main meal of the day (Humalog Mix 25, Humalog Mix 50 or Novomix 30). When Lantus was first introduced, NICE gave the following guidelines for its use in type 2 patients:

- those who require assistance from a carer or healthcare professional to administer injections
- those whose lifestyle is significantly restricted by recurrent symptomatic hypoglycaemic episodes
- those who would otherwise need twice-daily basal injections in combination with oral hypoglycaemia drugs.

However, as Lantus has a lower risk of nocturnal hypoglycaemia than NPH intermediate insulin, it is commonly used in this regimen, especially as it specifically has a licence for use with oral hypoglycaemia agents (Yki-Järvinen *et al.*, 2000).

The patient injects once a day at the appropriate time and tests the pre-breakfast blood glucose (there is no need for them to check at other times unless they feel hypoglycaemic or unwell). They increase the dose of insulin by small increments (e.g. by 2 units) every three days until the pre-breakfast insulin is in the target range most mornings (between 4 and 6 mmol/l). Depending on the degree of insulin resistance (usually related to weight), some patients may need relatively large doses of insulin, and they will need encouragement to keep titrating up the dose of insulin until they reach target.

This is a very simple regimen to initiate and, given a clear target to reach and a simple algorithm to follow, most patients can self-titrate the insulin dose appropriately. The AT.LANTUS (A Trial comparing LAntus algorithms to achieve Normal blood glucose Targets in Uncontrolled blood Sugar) study compared patients who were advised weekly by their healthcare professional which insulin dose to have according to their blood glucose results, and patients who self-titrated their insulin using this simple algorithm. The study demonstrated that the latter actually achieved a lower HbA1c with no increase in hypoglycaemia (Davies *et al.*, 2005).

Once the pre-breakfast target is reached, the patient should then vary the timing of their daily blood glucose test to ensure the blood glucose is in single figures most of the day. If the patient describes symptoms of hypoglycaemia in the day as they build up the insulin dose, or the patient's HbA1c is < 8% when initiating insulin, the dose of oral hypoglycaemic agent can be reduced or even discontinued as the fasting target is approached.

Many patients will be able to reach an HbA1c of 7% or less on this regimen. However, as their beta cell failure progresses over time, they will need to increase their insulin dose gradually to maintain the target pre-breakfast test, and they will notice it is more difficult to achieve normal blood sugar readings during the day. Patients starting on this regimen, therefore, should be warned that they will require additional insulin injections in the future.

As this regimen will only meet basal insulin requirements, it is not suitable for patients with type 1 diabetes unless they are elderly and frail or in other circumstances where tight control is not an advantage for the patient.

Basal plus

The basal plus regimen is a simple method to introduce a basal bolus regimen to patients with type 2 diabetes regimen who cannot maintain normal blood sugars after one or more meals despite achieving normal pre-breakfast blood sugar readings with a basal insulin. The patient continues with the basal insulin dose that keeps their pre-breakfast blood sugar in target. They vary the times of their daily blood glucose tests and check their blood sugar 2 hours after breakfast or lunch or evening meal in order to identify which meal(s) causes their blood sugar to rise above target. Often patients find it is just after the main meal of the day that the blood glucose rises to 10 mmol/l or higher.

The patient then adds a small dose (e.g. 4 units) of rapid-acting or soluble insulin before that meal. By testing their blood glucose 2 hours after the meal, they can gradually adjust the mealtime insulin dose until the glucose levels are in single figures. If the content of the main meal varies, patients may learn that certain carbohydrate-dense meals (e.g. pasta-based) will require a bigger dose of insulin than a meal with less carbohydrate). The advantage of this regimen is that the patient can vary when they have the mealtime insulin, depending on what time of day they have their main meal (e.g. in the evening in the week and at lunchtime on Sunday).

Twice daily regimen

The insulin mixtures are usually used twice daily. They provide a basal component and a short- or rapid-acting component in a fixed proportion. Although this regimen has the advantage of providing some mealtime cover with only two injections a day, the fixed mix means that patients need to eat regularly and have similar carbohydrate portions with their meals each day. The mixtures that include a rapid-acting analogue can be taken immediately before or just after the meal. Mixtures using soluble insulin should be taken about 20 minutes before meals. As they are a mixture of two insulins, patients should be advised to resuspend the insulin thoroughly before each injection.

When starting patients on this regimen, a small dose is given at breakfast (e.g. 12 units) and with the evening meal. Blood glucose tests during the day (i.e. 2 hours after breakfast, before lunch, mid-afternoon and before the evening injection) demonstrate the effectiveness of the morning injection. The dose can be increased gradually (e.g. by 10% every few days) until these tests are within the target range most of the time. Conversely, the dose is decreased by the same amount if the tests in the day are falling frequently below 4 mmol/l. Tests during the evening, before bed, during the night and before breakfast inform the patient whether the evening dose is correct. The insulin dose is adjusted up or down by 10% as appropriate.

Basal bolus regimen

The basal bolus regimen aims to mimic the insulin production of the individual without diabetes and is the regimen of choice for someone with type 1 diabetes and for patients with type 2 diabetes with very little residual beta cell function. It is also useful for any patient who has variable meal times and meal sizes, as the mealtime insulin is given whenever the meal is taken, rather than the patient having to eat at regular times to fit in with the insulin regimen.

The basal insulin is adjusted until the pre-breakfast blood glucose is within the normal range (ideally between 4 and 6 mmol/l most of the time for most patients). A small dose of rapid-acting analogue (or soluble insulin can also be used if additional basal insulin is required during the day, despite normal pre-breakfast glucose readings) is injected before each meal, whenever the patient decides to eat. Comparing the blood glucose readings before and 2 hours after the injection and meal will inform the patient about the effectiveness of the dose given. If the postprandial test is lower than the preprandial test, then too much insulin was given with that meal. Conversely, if the postprandial blood glucose test is much higher than the preprandial test, then insufficient insulin was given for that meal. Patients can learn to adjust each mealtime insulin until the pre- and postprandial blood glucose tests are similar.

Managing insulin therapy in the individual

Even though insulins are becoming more sophisticated, and the use of multiple injections in the basal bolus regimen aims to mimic normal insulin production, insulin-replacement therapy is still a crude mimic of the fine balance between insulin, prevailing blood glucose and other hormones and environmental factors that a person without diabetes achieves automatically. Being able to achieve glycaemia as near normal as possible without disabling hypoglycaemia requires a considerable amount of support and education. A structured education programme for patients with type 1 diabetes is available in a number of centres across the UK to empower people to manage intensive insulin therapy more effectively. The course (Dose Adjustment for Normal Eating: DAFNE) involves a week in which a diabetes specialist nurse and a dietitian support a maximum of eight patients with type 1 diabetes. A randomised control trial showed that this approach improved quality of life and glycaemic control in 169 people with type 1 diabetes (DAFNE Study Group, 2002)

Although there is not similar evidence available for type 2 diabetes, patients using a basal bolus regimen should still have some understanding about the effect of the carbohydrate content of their meals on their blood glucose levels. They can then make appropriate adjustments between meals (e.g. a carbohydrate-dense pasta-based meal will require a bigger dose of insulin than a plate of meat, vegetables and a few boiled new potatoes). Also, it is important that patients with type 2 diabetes, who are usually overweight, do not 'eat for their insulin' and that if they are not hungry and want to omit a meal, they should omit that mealtime insulin.

The three case studies (Boxes 6.2–6.4) illustrate how different patients require varying insulins and regimens. Some patients will need specialist care (Box 6.5).

Box 6.2 Susan, aged 19, student with type 1 diabetes

Regimen: Levemir at breakfast and at bedtime with Novorapid with each meal.

Susan has had type 1 diabetes since she was 8 years old. She produces no insulin herself at all and is completely dependent on the insulin she injects daily. She, therefore, needs an insulin regimen that mimics how her body used to produce insulin. She needs a long-acting 'background' insulin that keeps her fasting blood sugars within the normal range, and rapid-acting insulin with meals to prevent her blood sugar from rising too quickly after meals.

By learning how the quantity of carbohydrate in her meals affects her blood sugar levels, she can learn to adjust the dose of her mealtime insulin according to what she wants to eat. Using the rapid-acting analogue insulins with meals, in addition to a basal insulin, she injects whenever she wants to eat so this allows her to keep good control of her blood sugar despite eating irregularly and sleeping late in the mornings!

Box 6.3 Joan, aged 85, lives alone and has type 2 diabetes

Regimen: Lantus daily given mid morning by a district nurse.

Joan has had type 2 diabetes for 10 years. She still produces insulin but not enough to keep her blood sugar in the normal range. She initially controlled her blood sugar by improving her diet but after a year needed metformin and then had gliclazide added in. After seven years, despite maximum doses of both drugs, her HbA1c was 9%. A daily dose of 10 units of Lantus was added to her oral therapy (and her own remaining insulin production). This dose was titrated every few days until her fasting blood sugar was usually approximately 6 mmol/l. As Lantus is absorbed slowly and fairly evenly over 24 hours, the insulin can be given at a time that is convenient to Joan and the district nursing team, rather than related to meals. Joan is elderly and lives alone, so symptom control with avoidance of hypoglycaemia is the main aim of her treatment.

Box 6.4 Roger aged 53, office worker, with type 2 diabetes

Regimen: Humalog Mix 25 twice a day (with breakfast and evening meal)

Roger has had type 2 diabetes for six years, controlled for four years with metformin, gliclazide and recently pioglitazone. As his HbA1c gradually increased to 8.1% despite his best efforts with diet and exercise, his GP advised that he should add in insulin. A daily dose of 10 units of Lantus was started. He continued with the gliclazide and metformin but the pioglitazone was discontinued because the use of glitazones with insulin was contraindicated at that time. Roger checked his blood sugar before breakfast each morning and increased the dose by 2 units every three days until his fasting blood sugar was between 4 and 6 mmol/l. However, he noticed his blood sugars after meals were rising to double figures. He did not want to inject with every meal, so he decided to change to a twice-daily insulin mixture, which gave him a background insulin with a bolus of rapid-acting insulin with breakfast and evening meal. His gliclazide was discontinued but he continued with the metformin as this improves his insulin sensitivity. Twice-daily mixtures need to be given before breakfast and evening meals at regular times, but as he has a regular lifestyle, this is not a problem. He also has the option of adding in a midday injection for large Sunday lunches!

Box 6.5 Who needs specialist referral?

- Patients transferring from animal to human-identical or analogue insulins.
- Patients who have needle phobia and who may benefit from using the MHI-500 or SQ-Pen needle-free device (see Fig. 6.9, below; although these are available on prescription, patients may need considerable support in learning how to use these devices successfully)
- Patients who meet the criteria for an insulin pump
- Patients with type 1 diabetes who have persistently high pre-breakfast tests but have hypoglycaemia if their basal insulin is increased (an insulin pump may be beneficial)
- Patients with newly diagnosed type 1 diabetes
- Patients who have frequent episodes of disabling hypoglycaemia or diabetic ketoacidosis.

Adjusting insulin within a regimen

Most patients should be encouraged to monitor their blood glucose if they are using insulin, and they should be taught how to adjust their insulin appropriately in relation to these tests (Table 6.9) and for variations in physical activity, meal size and other factors such as illness.

Insulin devices

Traditionally, patients requiring insulin needed to learn how to draw insulin from a vial with a syringe. This required a reasonable level of manual dexterity and adequate vision, and patients who did not possess these often then became dependent on carers or district nurses to inject their insulin. Some patients still prefer to use a syringe, and 1 ml syringes are useful for delivering large doses of insulin (up to 100 units) in a single injection (Fig. 6.1).

Most insulins are now available in disposable pens, or in 3 ml cartridges that fit a particular pen device, and patients starting insulin therapy should be taught how to use an insulin device of their choice. Disposable devices come in boxes of five pens, each containing 3 ml of insulin (i.e. 300 units) (Fig. 6.2). As the name suggests, when the pen is empty, the whole device is thrown away in household rubbish, once the needle has been safely disposed of. Cartridges are inserted into a reusable pen (available on prescription) in a similar way to using a fountain pen. When the cartridge is empty, the cartridge is replaced. Patients should always keep a spare pen available in case of breakage or malfunction. Reusable pens are usually specific to the make of insulin (Fig. 6.3). For example, the Humapen Luxura pen, produced by Lilly, will only accept 3 ml cartridges of insulin produced by Lilly, and the Novopen, produced by Novo Nordisk, can only be used with Novo Nordisk insulin cartridges. The Autopen

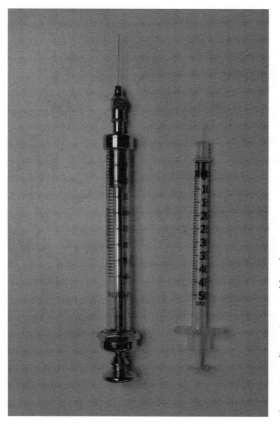

Fig. 6.1 Insulin syringes: old and new.

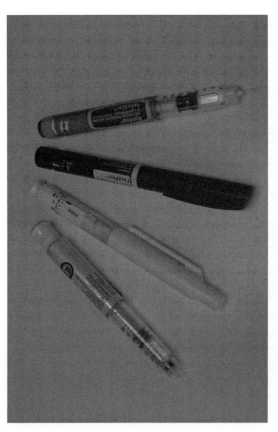

Fig. 6.2 Disposable insulin pen devices. From left to right: disposable pen by Lilly, Optiset by Sanofi Aventis, Flexpen by Novo Nordisk, and Solostar by Sanofi Aventis.

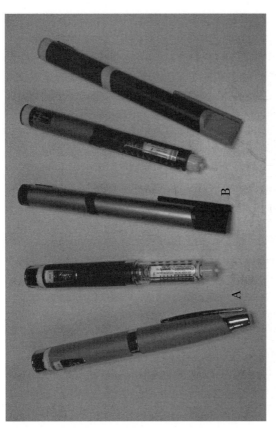

Fig. 6.3 Refillable insulin pen devices. A, Novopen by Novo Nordisk; B, Humapen Luxura by Lilly.

produced by Owen Mumford can be used for cartridges of animal insulin produced by Wockhardt and the Lilly insulin cartridges, whereas the Autopen 24 is specified for Sanofi-Aventis insulin cartridges.

Some devices have particular features which may be useful for certain patients. The InnoLet device, produced by Novo Nordisk for their Levemir, Mixtard 30 and Insulatard range, looks like an egg timer with a large dial and may be useful for those with manual dexterity problems or poor eyesight (Fig. 6.4). The Opiset pen can be preset, which is useful for people on a stable daily dose of insulin who have poor vision (Fig. 6.5). The OptiClik pen can be dialled up to a dose of 80 units, which is useful for people requiring large doses of insulin (Fig. 6.5). The plunger length does not vary with dose size, which may be helpful for people with manual dexterity problems who need to inject large doses. However, this pen is not currently available on prescription but it can be obtained through the manufacturers, Sanofi- Aventis (01483 505515). The Autopen Classic and Autopen 24 devices have attachments to facilitate easier dose dialling and depressing the plunger, which may also be helpful for people with manual dexterity problems (Fig. 6.6).

Insulin pen needles are available from various manufacturers and range in size from 5 to 12.7 mm. Most people find a 6 or 8 mm suitable. Patients should be advised to use a new needle for every injection as microscopic damage occurs to the end of the needle when it is used.

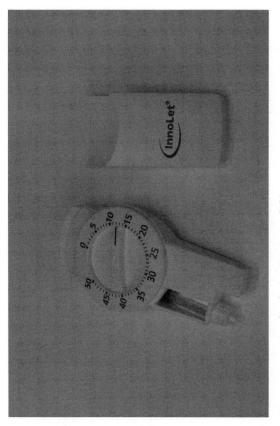

Fig. 6.4 InnoLet insulin device (Novo Nordisk).

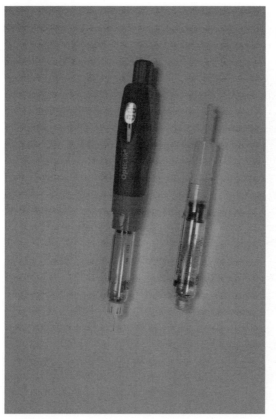

Fig. 6.5 Opticlik pen device showing pen device and cartridge (Sanofi Aventis).

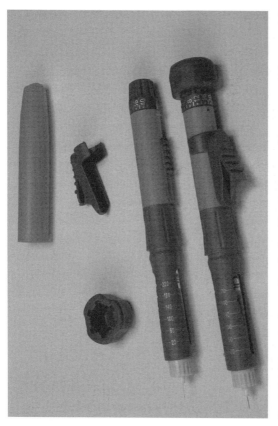

Fig. 6.6 Autopen by Owen Mumford, with attachments for patients with manual dexterity problems.

Vials and syringes should still be used by district nurses giving insulin to dependent patients, as there is a lower risk of needle stick injury with syringes than removing needles from insulin devices. However, if healthcare professionals do need to use an insulin pen to give insulin to a patient (e.g. because the patient requires an insulin that is not available in vials, such as Novomix 30), the Autocover needles, produced by Novo Nordisk, could be used. The needles are so designed that they are sheathed throughout the complete injection and cannot be used more than once (Fig. 6.7). As the needle is never exposed, they may also be helpful for patients with needle phobia. Novo Nordisk also provide a needle-removing device, which is useful for healthcare professionals supporting patients using an insulin pen; it allows conventional needles to be removed safely until the patient is able to do this themselves (Fig. 6.8; contact Novo Nordisk 0845 6005055).

Needle-free devices are also available for patients who have needle phobia (Fig. 6.9).

Inhaled insulin

Inhaled insulin was available for a short period in 2007 but was commercially unviable and so was withdrawn by the manufacturers (Pfizer) at the end of 2007. It was similar in profile to mealtime injected insulin so a background insulin injection was still required for most patients. The insulin was available in 1 and 3 mg blisters,

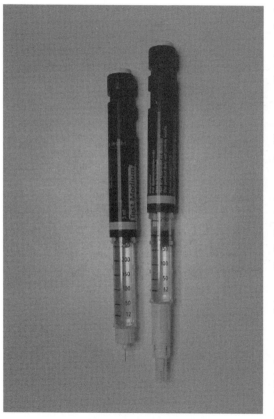

Fig. 6.7 Autocover safety needle (bottom) compared with a conventional needle (top).

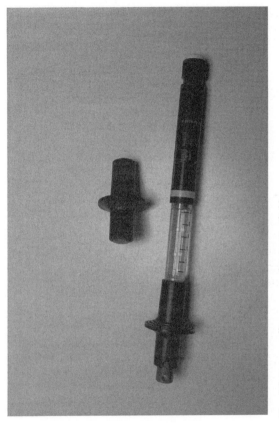

Fig. 6.8 Pen needle remover (Novo Nordisk).

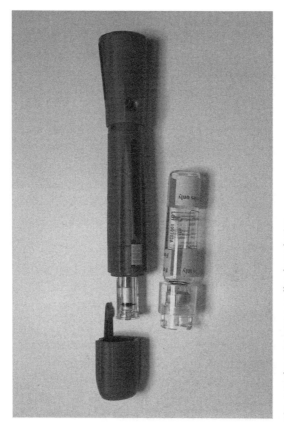

Fig. 6.9 The MHI-500 needles-less device.

not units: 1 mg was equivalent to 3 units but 3 mg was equivalent to 8 units of injected insulin. The device required a reasonable degree of manual dexterity (Fig. 6.10). The NICE guidance stated it should not be recommended for routine treatment of type 1 and 2 diabetes, but it might be useful as a treatment option for people who have poor glycaemic control and have needle phobia or severe and persistent problems with injection sites (e.g. lipohypertrophy) (NICE, 2006). It was recommended that initiation should be managed at a specialist diabetes centre, and spirometry checks were required. Inhaled insulin is contraindicated in people who smoke or who have chronic lung conditions like asthma and chronic obstructive pulmonary disease. It may become available again through other manufacturers.

What all patients using insulin therapy need to know

Hypoglycaemia

Patients, and their close associates, should be aware of the signs and symptoms of hypoglycaemia, the potential causes of this, and how to treat it (see Chapter 7).

Possible causes of hypoglycaemia:

- too much insulin injected
- insufficient carbohydrate eaten for dose of insulin given

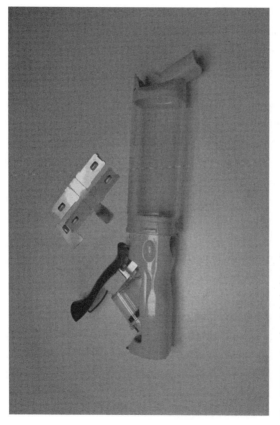

Fig. 6.10 Device for inhaled insulin.

- delayed meal (for those on fixed twice-daily regimens)
- alcohol use
- more physical activity than usual
- insulin injected into a muscle instead of subcutaneous fat.

Other causes of hypoglycaemia can include:

- progressive deterioration of renal function (so insulin half-life is extended, and regular injections become superimposed on each other)
- loss of weight without reduction of insulin dose
- addition of metformin (improves insulin sensitivity)
- reduction or withdrawal of agents that increase insulin resistance (e.g. steroids)
- early pregnancy
- changing from a lipohypertrophic injection site (see below).

Patients should be competent in setting up their insulin-delivery device and use the correct injection technique, into subcutaneous fat in a suitable area. The recommended sites for insulin injections are the buttocks, the abdomen and the top third of the thigh (front or side). Arms are not recommended for self-injection as most patients should 'pinch an inch' of fat with one hand while injecting with the other (Fig. 6.11). This is difficult to achieve in the arm but is suitable when the injection is being performed by someone else. It is important that

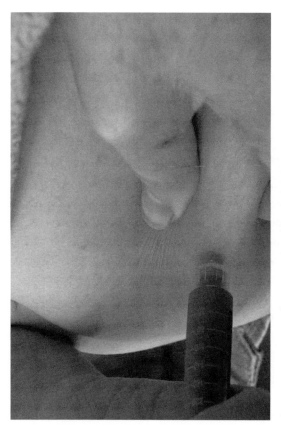

Fig. 6.11 Injecting insulin using a 'pinching-up' technique.

injection sites are varied as repeated injections in the same site over time lead to the development of lipohypertrophy. This presents as a firm fatty lump under the skin. Unfortunately, insulin injected into this area is absorbed at an erratic rate, leading to poor glycaemic control. Care needs to be taken when advising patients to avoid injecting into these sites as they may find that their blood glucose levels suddenly plummet as the insulin is absorbed properly from the new site.

Insulin storage

Insulin not in use should be stored in the fridge, but should not be frozen. Insulin in current use will last for about a month at room temperature, so it can be left in the bedroom for patients injecting at night, on the dining table or in a handbag, for example, for mealtime insulins, which may make it easier for patients to remember to inject at the correct time. When travelling abroad, insulin should be carried in the patient's hand luggage to avoid it getting frozen in the hold. Small cool-bags can be purchased from pharmacists or the Medical Shop for keeping insulin cool in hot countries.

Driving

Drivers should inform their insurers and the DVLA that they are using insulin. Driving licences should be renewed every three years, unless the patient has lost the symptoms of hypoglycaemia ('hypo unawareness') or their eyesight is not good enough. People using insulin are not allowed to hold HGV or PSV licences so this may be a reason why some patients, whose employment will be affected by this rule, may refuse to use insulin.

Episodes of ill health

Patients need to know what to do with their insulin during episodes of sickness and ailments such as influenza when they may have poor appetite. It is essential that they do not stop their insulin because they are not eating. This is a natural reaction, however, because patients may be concerned that they may become hypoglycaemic if they continue with their insulin but do not eat (indeed, they may have been informed that this a common cause of hypoglycaemia).

During illness or trauma, the body becomes more insulin resistant because of the release of counter-regulatory hormones, particularly cortisol. Blood glucose, therefore, often rises above normal, despite the patient not eating. Stopping insulin in the insulin-deficient patient will increase glucagon production and, therefore, gluconeogenesis and glycogenolysis by the liver, and in the case of patients with type 1 diabetes, lead to the development of diabetic ketoacidosis. The rule is quite clear for these people: NEVER STOP YOUR INSULIN. In fact, insulin doses often need to be increased during this time. Ketone testing (Chapter 4) is a useful guide to support this decision during periods of sickness.

In the patient with type 2 diabetes, the rules are not so clear cut, depending on the amount of relative insulin deficiency and the patient's usual calorie intake. Missing out meals may result in lower blood glucose levels than usual, despite the effect of illness. All patients, therefore, should be advised to monitor their blood glucose levels more closely during periods of illness, and to adjust their insulin doses as required (up or down by 10–20% if hyperglycaemic or hypoglycaemic).

REFERENCES

DAFNE Study Group (2002) Training in flexible, intensive insulin management to enable dietary freedom in people with type 1 diabetes: Dose Adjustment for Normal Eating (DAFNE) randomised controlled trial. *British Medical Journal* **325**: 746–59.

Davies M., Storms F., Shutler S. *et al.* (2005) Improvement of glycaemic control in subjects with poorly controlled type 2 diabetes. *Diabetes Care* **28**: 1282–8.

Yki-Järvinen H., Dressler A. and Ziemen M. (2000) Less nocturnal hypoglycemia and better post-dinner glucose control with bedtime insulin glargine compared with bedtime NPH insulin during insulin combination therapy in type 2 diabetes. HOE 901/3002 Study Group. *Diabetes Care* **23**: 1130–6.

RELEVANT NICE GUIDELINES

Diabetes (types 1 and 2): long acting insulin analogues.
Technology Appraisal No. 53, December 2002.

Diabetes (type 1): insulin pump therapy.
Technology Appraisal No. 57, February 2003 (currently
being reviewed).

Diagnosis and management of type 1 diabetes in
children, young people and adults. *Clinical Guidance*
No. 15, July 2004.

Diabetes (type 1 and 2): inhaled insulin. *Technology
Appraisal* No. 113, December 2006.

MEDICAL SUPPLIER

Medical shop
Freepost 0F1727, Woodstock, Oxon OX20 1BR
Freephone: 0800 731 6959
www.medicalshop.co.uk

Chapter 7

Management of increased cardiovascular risk

Traditionally, the management of both type 1 and type 2 diabetes has been focused on glycaemic control. However, particularly in type 2 diabetes, these patients are at very much increased cardiovascular risk, which is illustrated by the observation by Haffner *et al.* (1998) that someone with type 2 diabetes has a similar risk of having a myocardial infarction as someone without diabetes who has already had a myocardial infarction. Life expectancy of someone with type 2 diabetes, if diagnosed between 40 and 60 years of age, is reduced by about 5–10 years. Mortality rate is increased more than twofold; fatal coronary heart disease is increased two- to fourfold; fatal stroke is increased two- to threefold; coronary heart disease is increased two- to threefold; cerebrovascular disease is increased more than twofold; peripheral vascular disease is increased two- to threefold; and cardiac failure is increased two- to fivefold (Krentz and Bailey, 2001).

These greatly increased risks in type 2 diabetes result from the clustering of risk factors seen in patients with this condition, particularly hypertension and dyslipidaemia. The UK Prospective Diabetes Study (UKPDS) Group (1998) showed that improved blood glucose had relatively little impact on the incidence of cardiovascular complications, but reducing blood pressure reduced risk significantly for these complications.

The Steno-2 study (Gaede *et al.*, 2003) demonstrated that a multifactorial approach to target all major risk factors resulted in a much greater reduction in cardiovascular endpoints. A group of 160 patients in Denmark who had type 2 diabetes and microalbuminuria were randomised to conventional or intensive treatment. The latter included management of hyperglycaemia, hypertension, dyslipidaemia, encouraging smoking cessation and use of aspirin, and it resulted in a 50% reduction in the incidence of cardiovascular events. Non-fatal myocardial infarction was reduced by 70%, non-fatal stroke by 85% and amputations by 50%. This holistic, integrated approach to management of diabetes is now commonplace, and patients are being encouraged, in addition to adopting healthy lifestyle changes to improve weight and physical activity levels, to 'know their numbers' in controlling all aspects of their diabetes, not just the HbA1c.

Assessment of cardiovascular risk in diabetes

The following should be performed at diagnosis and at least annually from then on:

- current or previous cardiovascular disease
- age
- family history of premature cardiovascular disease
- body mass index

- abdominal adiposity
- smoking status
- blood pressure
- lipid profile
- albumin excretion rate
- presence of atrial fibrillation (for stroke).

Risk equations developed for people without diabetes should not be used.

Dyslipidaemia

Non-pharmacological interventions to improve the lipid profile

The typical lipid profile of the patient with type 2 diabetes includes hypertriglyceridaemia, low levels of protective HDL-cholesterol, with raised levels of atherogenic small dense low density lipoprotein (LDL)-cholesterol and total cholesterol. The management of dyslipidaemia involves lowering levels of harmful cholesterol without further lowering HDL-cholesterol, but ideally increasing it as HDL-cholesterol has a cardioprotective effect. It takes up cholesterol esters from the peripheral tissues when cells are broken down, and removes these from the circulation by transferring them back to the liver.

Although the evidence supports statin treatment for most people with diabetes, no matter what their total cholesterol is, they should be used in addition to a healthy lifestyle. Aerobic physical exercise can be useful in reducing triglyceridaemia and LDL-cholesterol and raising HDL-cholesterol. Improving metabolic control by adding in insulin therapy may improve triglycerides, LDL-cholesterol and total cholesterol as hepatic LDL receptors (which are the major regulators of plasma LDL) are dependent on insulin. Reducing excess alcohol may be important as excessive alcohol can exacerbate hypertriglyceridaemia, but conversely moderate alcohol can increase HDL-cholesterol.

Attaining ideal body weight, reducing total fat intake to about 30% of total calorie intake, and saturated fat to less than 10% of the total daily calorie intake will also reduce triglycerides. Use of monounsaturated oils such as olive, pure vegetable and rapeseed oils increases HDL-cholesterol. Polyunsaturated oils such as sunflower oils will lower LDL-cholesterol but unfortunately can lower HDL-cholesterol too, but they are preferable to saturated fats like butter or lard. Smoking cessation has the added benefit of increasing HDL-cholesterol by up to 10%.

Table 7.1 gives the target guidelines for blood lipids. Excluding other causes of dyslipidaemia, such as hepatic dysfunction, renal impairment and, more commonly, hypothyroidism, is important.

Pharmacological options for managing dyslipidaemia

There are a number of medications in use for addressing the dyslipidaemia seen in diabetes. As people with

Table 7.1 Management of dyslipidaemia
(NICE and JBS 2)

Lipid	Target (mmol/l)
Total cholesterol	4 or less
LDL	$<2\,mmol/l^{a}$
HDL	>1.0
Triglycerides	$<1.7^{a}$

LDL, low density lipoprotein; HDL, high density
lipoprotein.
[a] Targets recommended by the Joint British
  Societies guidelines in JBS 2 (2005).

diabetes are at such high cardiovascular risk, the Joint
British Societies guidelines (2005) (JBS 2; Box 7.1) on
prevention of cardiovascular disease in clinical practice
recommend that it is not necessary to use risk scores
on these patients and that all patients with type 1 and
type 2 diabetes over the age of 40 should receive statin
therapy.

Consequently, statins are the first-line therapy in these
adults, because the evidence base for their effectiveness is
so strong. Table 7.2 summarises the treatment options.

Statin therapy

Lipid lowering is the most effective single intervention to
reduce cardiovascular risk in people with diabetes. There
are two large clinical trials that have provided the evidence
for this (Box 7.2).

Table 7.2 Summary of the treatments for dyslipidaemia

Drug	Effect
Statins	Reduce LDL
	Small reductions in triglycerides
	Slight increase in HDL (5–10%)
Fibrates	Reduce triglycerides by up to 50%
	Increase HDL by up to 20%
Nicotinic acid	Reduces triglycerides by approximately 40–50%
	Reduces LDL by up to 20%
	Increases HDL by up to 30%
Omega-3 fish oils	Reduces triglycerides
Ezetimibe	Reduces LDL, especially in combination with a statin

LDL, low density lipoprotein; HDL, high density lipoprotein.

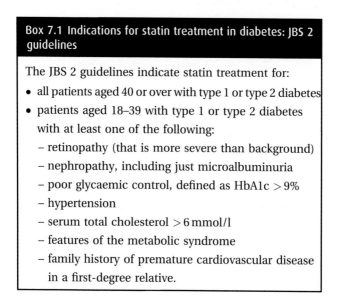

Box 7.1 Indications for statin treatment in diabetes: JBS 2 guidelines

The JBS 2 guidelines indicate statin treatment for:

- all patients aged 40 or over with type 1 or type 2 diabetes
- patients aged 18–39 with type 1 or type 2 diabetes with at least one of the following:
  - retinopathy (that is more severe than background)
  - nephropathy, including just microalbuminuria
  - poor glycaemic control, defined as HbA1c > 9%
  - hypertension
  - serum total cholesterol > 6 mmol/l
  - features of the metabolic syndrome
  - family history of premature cardiovascular disease in a first-degree relative.

Box 7.2 Trials of lipid-lowering therapy in diabetes

The Heart Protection Study (HPS) (Collins *et al.*, 2002)

This was a randomised prospective placebo-controlled trial involving 5963 adults between 40 and 80 years who had either type 1 or type 2 diabetes, with an additional 14 573 people with occlusive arterial disease but no diabetes. They were randomised to receive either 40 mg simvastatin or placebo daily, and followed for five years. In the treatment group, major cardiovascular events were reduced by 24%.

The Collaborative AtoRvastatin Diabetes Study (CARDS) (Colhourn *et al.*, 2004)

This trial comprised 2838 patients with type 2 diabetes and at least one other cardiac risk factor (defined as smoking, hypertension, retinopathy, microalbuminuria or proteinuria). Patients were randomised to either atorvastatin 10 mg daily or placebo. The trial was terminated early as the beneficial effects of the statin in reducing stroke so dramatically made it unethical to continue with placebo. The treated group had a 36% reduction in coronary events and a 48% reduction in stroke compared with placebo.

Table 7.3 Statins currently available in the UK

Drug name	Starting dose (mg/day)	Maximum dose (mg/day)
Atorvastatin (Lipitor)	10	80
Fluvastatin	40	80
Pravastatin	10	40
Rosuvastatin (Crestor)	5–10	40 (requires specialist supervision; this high dose is contraindicated in Asian patients)
Simvastatin	10	80

NICE have recently updated their guidelines to reflect the recommendations of JBS 2. There are a number of statins available (Table 7.3) and all have the same mode of action. The drugs are competitive inhibitors of the enzyme 3-hydroxy-3-methylglutaryl coenzyme A (HMG-CoA) reductase, an enzyme involved in cholesterol synthesis in the liver. The reduction of cholesterol then leads to increasing number of LDL receptors on cell surfaces, which increases the clearance of LDL from the circulation. Statins, therefore, reduce total cholesterol and LDL-cholesterol in the bloodstream. They may also have a small effect on increasing the protective HDL-cholesterol.

Pharmacokinetics.   Statins are well absorbed from the gastrointestinal tract. As the cholesterol pathway occurs during sleep, statins should be taken orally at bedtime.

Contraindications. Statins are contraindicated in patients with active liver disease or unexplained persistent elevations in serum transaminases, severe renal impairment, myopathy, concomitant ciclosporin therapy, pregnancy and breast-feeding, and women of child-bearing age who are not using contraception (in case they become pregnant). Rosuvastatin, at the highest dose of 40 mg, is contraindicated in South Asian patients.

Caution. Statins interact with several other drugs commonly used in patients with diabetes, including fibrates, and also grapefruit juice. Use with concomitant fibrates should be managed by specialist care. Patients with predisposing factors for developing myopathy or rhabdomyolysis should be monitored closely.

Side-effects. Headache, altered liver function, gastrointestinal effects including abdominal pain, flatulence, diarrhoea/ constipation, nausea and vomiting, dizziness can all occur. Rash and hypersensitivity reactions are rare. Muscle effects such as myalgia, myositis and myopathy may occur. If muscle symptoms are severe or serum creatine kinase levels are raised to more than five times the normal limit, then the statin should be discontinued. Rhabdomyolysis is very rare.

Monitoring. Patients taking statins should be questioned for symptoms of unexplained muscle pain, tenderness and weakness, and serum creatine kinase should be measured to rule out adverse effects. Patients taking statins should be advised to report these symptoms immediately. Liver function should be assessed annually, and statins discontinued if transaminases rise to more than three times the upper limit of normal.

Fibrates

Fibrates increase HDL-cholesterol and reduce triglycerides, and they are recommended when these are abnormal but total cholesterol is normal. They are PPAR-alpha agonists and work by stimulating lipoprotein lipase, which results in an increase in hydrolysis of triglyceride in chylomicrons and VLDL particles. They also liberate free fatty acid for storage in fat or for metabolism in striated muscle. Unfortunately, the Fenofibrate Intervention and Event Lowering in Diabetes (FIELD) study showed a non-significant reduction in cardiovascular events when testing fenofibrate against placebo (Keech *et al.*, 2005). The role of fibrates, therefore, remains uncertain, despite their actions appearing to tackle the key characteristics seen in people with diabetes. They are recommended if the fasting triglyceride level is > 1.7 mmol/l, once LDL-cholesterol is as optimally controlled as possible.

Fibrates currently available in the UK include:

- bezafibrate
- ciprofibrate
- fenofibrate
- gemfibrozil.

Contraindications. Fibrates should not be used in patients with hepatic insufficiency including biliary cirrhosis, severe renal impairment or gallbladder disease. They should be discontinued if plasma aspartate or alanine transaminase increases to more than three times the upper limit of normal. They must be avoided during pregnancy, and while breast-feeding.

Caution. High alcohol intake in conjunction with fibrates makes patients more prone to muscle side-effects. Patients with mild and moderate renal impairment and hypothyroidism should only use fibrates if monitored. Various fibrates interact with other drugs commonly used in people with diabetes such as anticoagulants, oral hypoglycaemic agents (repaglinide and rosiglitazone) and statins.

Side-effects. Fibrates can cause abdominal pain, nausea, diarrhoea, flatulence, erectile dysfunction and moderate rises in serum transaminases, Rarely, they can cause pancreatitis, muscle toxicity (myalgia, myositis, muscular cramps and weakness, and marked increases in plasma creatine phosphokinase); they should be discontinued if plasma creatine phosphokinase is greater than five times the normal level. They should also be discontinued if plasma transaminases increase to more than three times the upper limit of normal range.

Refer to specialist. Combination therapy with statins and fibrates should only be considered specialist care, as the risk of myopathy and rhabdomyolysis is greatly increased. Women who are planning a pregnancy and who are taking medications for dyslipidaemia should also receive specialist care.

Other agents for dyslipidaemia

The evidence base for other lipid-lowering agents is weaker than for statins and fibrates, and they are comparatively expensive. They are usually reserved for hyperlipidaemia that is not controlled with first-line drugs, or when there is intolerance to these.

Ezetimibe.   This agent is an inhibitor of intestinal cholesterol absorption. It can used as monotherapy, or more usually in combination with a statin to potentiate the action of the latter. A fixed combination of ezetimibe and simvastatin (10/40 mg) may be useful if the patient is concerned about the number of tablets to be taken.

Nicotinic acid (niacin) preparations.   Nicotinic acid is a vitamin and can be described as a broad-spectrum lipid-modifying agent because it is effective in raising HDL-cholesterol and reducing LDL-cholesterol and triglyceride levels. It can reduce insulin sensitivity and, therefore, may cause a deterioration in glycaemic control if used at high dosage in patients with insulin resistance. Facial flushing, palpitations and gastrointestinal disturbances can be more of a problem, and these are the reasons why many patients cannot tolerate them, although the once-daily, slow-release agent Niaspan has a much lower side-effect profile. Niacin is usually used in combination with a statin.

Omega-3 fatty acids. Omega-3 fish oils reduce plasma triglycerides by a process that is not fully understood, but they also increase cholesterol. They are rich in a number of highly unsaturated fatty acids that have other potentially important effects such as inhibition of platelet function, prolongation of bleeding time, anti-inflammatory effects and reduction of plasma fibrinogen. This may account for their effect of reducing ischaemic heart disease. They can be taken as monotherapy or in combination with statins.

Hypertension

Between 50 and 80% of people with type 2 diabetes have hypertension, as defined by a blood pressure greater than 140/90. Approximately 80% of all people with type 2 diabetes also die prematurely from cardiovascular disease. Reducing blood pressure reduces the risk of microvascular and macrovascular complications and is the most important factor in preventing diabetic nephropathy and end-stage renal failure. (It has been estimated that the time from the first positive protein urine strip result to kidney failure is about nine years. This time interval can be doubled through appropriate treatment of blood pressure.)

Trial data show that the greater the blood pressure reduction, the greater the benefit, with no blood pressure threshold below which risk declines no further. Evidence from the UK Prospective Diabetes Study (Holman *et al.*, 1998; UKPDS, 1998; Box 7.3) shows that it is very important to lower blood pressure; that it does not appear to matter which agent is used; and that control of hypertension in people with diabetes is difficult and will require more than one agent in most cases.

Therapy should be started in patients who have had three separate blood pressure recordings of greater than 140/90 and who have been given non-pharmacological advice. The Joint British Societies (JBS 2) proposed an optimal target of 130/80 and NICE have proposed less than 140/80, but this should be 135/75 or less in patients with microalbuminuria or proteinuria. Control of hypertension in people with diabetes is notoriously difficult, but any reduction will have benefits. The magnitude of overall risk reduction is greater in patients with diabetes compared with people without diabetes, reflecting the higher absolute risk of cardiovascular disease in the diabetes population. Most patients will require a number of antihypertensive agents, which can mean there may be a problem with compliance, particularly as patients generally do not feel unwell with high blood pressure and, therefore, may not see the benefits of taking so many tablets.

Box 7.3 The UK Prospective Diabetes Studies on diabetes and blood pressure

UKPDS 38

Patients with type 2 diabetes with hypertension were allocated to either tight control of blood pressure (758), using either an angiotensin-converting enzyme inhibitor (400) or a beta blocker (358), or less tight control (390). Patients were followed over eight years. Mean blood pressure was significantly reduced to a mean of 144/82 in the tightly controlled group compared with the less tightly controlled group (154/87; $p < 0.0001$).

There was a reduction in risk in the tight control group of 24% in any diabetes endpoints, 44% in strokes, 56% in heart failure and 37% for microvascular endpoints (particularly retinopathy).

UKPDS 39

This trial looked at whether the angiotensin-converting enzyme inhibitor used in the UKPDS 38 trial (captopril) or a beta blocker (atenolol) had a specific advantage in reducing microvascular or macrovascular complications of type 2 diabetes. The evidence showed that both were equally effective and safe in reducing blood pressure.

Assessment of the patient with hypertension

Secondary causes of hypertension should be excluded. These include:

- thyrotoxicosis
- acromegaly
- Cushing's syndrome
- phaeochromocytoma
- primary hyperparathyroidism.

Identify target organ damage:

- urinalysis to identify microalbuminuria or proteinuria (diabetic nephropathy)
- renal function and electrolytes (for renal impairment)
- electrocardiography for evidence of left ventricular hypertrophy and ischaemia.

Ambulatory blood pressure monitoring may be useful to identify 'white coat hypertension'.

Non-pharmacological strategies to control blood pressure

Lifestyle modification can reduce systolic blood pressure by 4–10 mmHg, which is as much as any antihypertensive drug. Measures include:

- weight reduction

- reducing salt intake (ideal levels are 6 g or less of sodium chloride per day); reducing the amount of processed foods and omitting adding salt at the table or in cooking will help to achieve this
- stopping smoking
- regular aerobic exercise
- reducing alcohol intake if heavy drinking
- stress management programme if appropriate.

Pharmacological options for managing hypertension

Although most patients with diabetes will require several antihypertensive agents, the British Hypertension Society and NICE recommend a stepwise approach to adding in medication, starting with an angiotensin-converting enzyme (ACE) inhibitor (or angiotensin-II receptor blocker, particularly if the ACE inhibitor is not tolerated) followed by a thiazide diuretic, then a calcium channel blocker then a beta blocker.

Therapy should be started in patients who have had three separate blood pressure recordings of greater than 140/90 and who have been given non-pharmacological advice.

Angiotensin-converting enzyme inhibitors
The ACE inhibitors are usually the first drug of choice in patients with diabetes because of their

Table 7.4 Recommended angiotensin-converting enzyme inhibitor dosage in treating hypertension

Drug	Starting daily dose (mg)	Maximum daily dosage (mg)
Captopril	25 (12.5 mg twice daily; 6.5 mg twice daily in the elderly)	100 (50 mg twice daily)
Cilazapril	1	5
Enalapril	5	40
Fosinopril	10	40
Imidapril	2.5	20
Lisinopril	5	80
Moexipril	3.75	15
Perindopril	4	8
Quinapril	10	80
Ramipril	1.25	10
Trandolapril	0.5	4

renoprotective effect. These agents act on the renin–angiotensin system by reducing the production of angiotensin II by the enzyme ACE. This has the effect of restricting the vasoconstriction caused by stimulation of the AT1 receptor. As ACE also promotes the breakdown of bradykinin, it is also known as bradykinase. Bradykinin has vasodilatory properties that also reduce blood pressure.

Table 7.4 gives the current recommended dosages for ACE inhibitors.

Side-effects. Because ACE inhibitors cause a build up of bradykinin, they produce a characteristic dry cough owing to its vasodilation effect in the lungs. They can also cause renal impairment, rash, pancreatitis and hyperkalaemia. Rarely, hypersensitivity results in facial and oral angioedema, in which case the ACE inhibitor should be stopped immediately.

Contraindications. The angiotensin system influences growth so inhibition of this system would affect fetal growth. Consequently, ACE inhibitors should not be used in pregnancy or in women contemplating pregnancy. They should not be used in renal artery stenosis as they can cause a rapid deterioration in renal function in patients with this condition.

Caution. All women of child-bearing age must be warned that they should not become pregnant when taking an ACE inhibitor, and they should seek preconception counselling when planning a pregnancy in order to change to a safer antihypertensive agent. Patients with peripheral vascular disease have a higher risk of renal artery stenosis so ACE inhibitors should be used with great caution in these patients.

Monitoring. Serum urea, electrolytes and creatinine should be checked immediately before and within 7 to 10 days of starting an ACE inhibitor, as a marked increase in creatinine usually indicates the presence

Table 7.5 Recommended angiotensin-II receptor blocker dosage for treating hypertension

Drug	Starting daily dose (mg)	Maximum daily dose (mg)
Candesartan	8	32
Eprosartan	600 (300 in patients over 75 years)	800
Irbesartan	150	300
Losartan	50	100
Olmesartan (Olmetec)	10	40
Telisartan (Micardis)	40	80
Valsartan	80	160

of renal artery stenosis. The blood test should be repeated after the same period after every increase in the dose.

Angiotensin-II receptor blockers

The angiotensin-II receptor blockers also act on the renin–angiotensin system but directly block the AT1 receptor lower down in the pathway and, therefore, do not cause a bradykinin build up with the resulting cough. There is good evidence of their renoprotective effects over and above their antihypertensive effects (Brenner *et al.*, 2001; Parving *et al.*, 2001; Box 7.4).

Table 7.5 lists the current recommended angiotensin-II receptor blockers used for treating hypertension.

Box 7.4 Studies on angiotensin-II receptor blockers

Irbesartan in MicroAlbuminuria in type II (IRMA II)

This was a multinational, randomised, double-blind, placebo-controlled study involving 590 patients with type 2 diabetes, hypertension and microalbuminuria. Patients were randomised to either daily iribesartan (150 or 300 mg) or placebo and followed for two years. Urinary albumin excretion rate significantly decreased in the iribesartan group, with restoration of normoalbuminuria occurring more in the group taking 300 mg iribesartan. The higher dose reduced the progression risk of diabetic nephropathy by 70%.

The Reduction of Endpoints in NIDDM with the Angiotensin II Antagonist Losartan study

In this study, 751 patients with type 2 diabetes and diabetic nephropathy were allocated to losartan and 762 were allocated to placebo and both groups were followed for approximately three years. Losartan reduced the incidence of a doubling of the serum creatinine concentration and end-stage renal disease but had no effect on the rate of death. This study demonstrated that losartan had positive effects on renal outcomes that were beyond its antihypertensive effect but that renal impairment should be identified and treated aggressively and early in its development.

Side-effects.   These drugs have relatively few side-effects but can cause hyperkalaemia, angioedema, rhinitis and pharyngitis.

Contraindications.   The angiotensin-II receptor blockers should not be used in pregnancy and renal artery stenosis, for the same reason given for ACE inhibitors.

Caution.   Women of child-bearing age should be warned not to conceive when using these agents. Patients with peripheral vascular disease are more likely to have renal artery stenosis. Urea and electrolytes should be measured 7–10 days after starting an angiotensin-II receptor blocker and after every increase in dose. A rapid rise in creatinine suggests the presence of renal artery stenosis and so the agent must be stopped immediately.

Thiazide diuretics

The thiazides are cheap, usually well tolerated, effective and work particularly well in combination with ACE inhibitors and angiotensin-II receptor blockers. They work to lower blood pressure by reducing sodium chloride and water retention. They are ineffective if renal function is significantly impaired (i.e. creatinine is greater than 150 µmol/l). The risk of worsened glycaemic control and dyslipidaemia that is seen with thiazide diuretics is minimal at low doses.

The most commonly used agent in this class is bendrofluazide (bendroflumethiazide) (2.5 mg daily).

Contraindications.   Bendrofluazide should not be used in patients with severe renal and hepatic impairment, hyponatraemia, hypercalcaemia, hypokalaemia or Addison's disease, or in women who are breast-feeding.

Side-effects.   These include electrolyte imbalance, postural hypotension, rash, hyperglycaemia, and impotence.

Use of aspirin

The National Service Framework for Diabetes, the Scottish Intercollegiate Guideline Network, and the NICE guidelines on managing blood pressure and lipids in people with diabetes (type 1 and 2) all recommend that for people with cardiovascular disease, aspirin 75 mg daily should be offered. There is currently no clear evidence of benefit of antiplatelet therapy for primary prevention in people with diabetes. The best evidence is from the Hypertension Optimal Treatment (HOT) trial (Hansson *et al.*, 1998; Box 7.5). The current recommendations of the American Diabetes Association (2006) is the use of aspirin in people aged over 40 years and those aged between 30 and 40 with additional cardiovascular risk factors. However, the JBS 2 guidelines (Joint British Societies, 2005) take a more cautious approach and suggest its use with:

- patients with established macrovascular disease
- patients aged 50 or over
- patients who are less than 50 and either have had diabetes for longer than 10 years or require treatment for hypertension.

Box 7.5 The Hypertension Optimal Treatment study

In this study, 18 790 patients aged between 50 and 80 years with hypertension (1501 with type 2 diabetes) were randomised to three different blood pressure targets; 9399 were randomised to take aspirin and 9391 placebo.

Aspirin reduced major cardiovascular events by 15% and myocardial infarction by 36% but had no effect on stroke. Although there was no difference in major bleeds between aspirin and placebo (7 and 8, respectively) there was significant difference between the two groups in non-fatal major bleeds (129 and 70, respectively; $p = < 0.001$).

Aspirin blocks prostaglandin synthetase action, which prevents formation of the platelet-aggregating substance thromboxane A_2 in the complex pathway of platelet activation. It is absorbed rapidly and has a duration of action of approximately 4–6 hours, and it is excreted by the kidneys.

Contraindications.   Aspirin should not be used in patients who are hypersensitive to salicylates, have a current or previous history of peptic ulceration, have severe hepatic or renal impairment, or have haemophila or other bleeding disorders. It should not be used in children under 16 years of age. It should also not be used in patients with uncontrolled hypertension (greater than 160 mmHg systolic pressure).

Caution. Patients with asthma may have an increased risk of salicylate sensitivity. Concurrent use with non-steroidal anti-inflammatory agents may increase the risk of gastrointestinal tract side-effects and bleeding. Use with warfarin also increases risk of bleeding.

Side-effects. Gastrointestinal upset, allergic reactions, bronchospasm, bleeding from the gastrointestinal tract can all occur.

Clopidogrel

This agent is at least as effective as aspirin but as it is much more expensive, it should only be used in people with aspirin intolerance. The risk of bleeding, which is a side-effect of aspirin is similar with this agent.

REFERENCES

American Diabetes Association (2006) Standards of medical care in diabetes in 2006. *Diabetes Care* **29**(Suppl. 1): S4–42.

Brenner B. M., Cooper M. E., de Zeeuw D. *et al.* (2001) The Reduction of Endpoints in NIDDM with the Angiotensin II Antagonist Losartan study (RENAAL). *New England Journal of Medicine* **345**: 861–9.

Colhourn H. M., Betteridge D. J., Durrington P. N. *et al.* (2004) Primary prevention of cardiovascular disease with atorvastatin in type 2 diabetes in the Collaborative AtoRvastatin Diabetes Study (CARDS): multicentre randomised placebo-controlled trial. *Lancet* **364**: 685–96.

Collins R., Armitage J., Parish S. *et al.* and the Heart Protection Study Collaborative Group (2002) MRC/BHF Heart Protection Study (HPS) of cholesterol-lowering with simvastatin in 5963 people with diabetes: a randomised placebo-controlled trial. *Lancet* **360**: 7–22.

Gaede P., Vedel P., Larsen N. Multifactorial intervention and cardiovascular disease in patients with type 2 diabetes. *New England Journal of Medicine* 2003 **348**: 383–93.

Haffner S. M., Lehto S., Ronnemaa T. *et al.* Mortality from coronary heart disease in subjects with type 2 diabetes and in nondiabetic subjects with and without prior myocardial infarction. *New England Journal of Medicine* 1998 **339**(4): 229–34.

Hansson L., Zanchetti A., Carruthers S. G. *et al.* (1998) Effects of intensive blood pressure lowering and low-dose aspirin in patients with hypertension: principal results of the Hypertension Optimal Treatment (HOT) randomised trial. *Lancet* **351**: 1755–62.

Holman R., Turner R., Stratton I. *et al.* (1998) Efficacy of atenolol and captopril in reducing risk of macrovascular and microvascular complications in type 2 diabetes: UKPDS 39. *British Medical Journal* **317**: 713–20.

Joint British Societies [British Cardiac Society, British Hypertension Society, Diabetes UK, HEART UK, Primary Care Cardiovascular Society, Stroke Association] (2005) JBS 2: Joint British Societies' guidelines on prevention of cardiovascular disease in clinical practice. *Heart* **91** (Suppl. V): v1–52.

Keech A., Simes R. J., Barter P. *et al.* Effects of long-term fenofibrate therapy on cardiovascular events in 9795 people with type 2 diabetes mellitus (the FIELD study): randomised controlled trial. *Lancet* **366** 2005: 1849–61.

Krentz A. J., and Bailey C. J. (2001) *Type 2 Diabetes in Practice*. London: Royal Society of Medicine Press.

Parving H. H., Lehnert H. and Mortensen J. B. (2001) Irbesartan in microalbuminuria in type II (IRMA II). *New England Journal of Medicine* **345**: 870–8.

UK Prospective Diabetes Study (UKPDS) Group (1998) Tight blood pressure (BP) control and risk of macrovascular complications in type 2 diabetes: UKPDS 38. *British Medical Journal* **317**: 703–11.

RELEVANT NICE GUIDELINE

Guideline on Statins for the Prevention of Cardiovascular Events. *Technology Appraisal* No. 94, January 2006.

Management of type 2 diabetes is currently being revised; publication expected in summer 2008.

Chapter 8

Acute and long-term complications

Hypoglycaemia

In the individual without diabetes, blood glucose rarely falls below the lower levels of the normal range, even during periods of fasting. This is achieved by a number of interactions between insulin, glucagon and the liver, as described in Chapter 3. However, patients taking hypoglycaemic agents that stimulate the beta cells (sulphonylureas and the prandial regulators), or who are using insulin therapy, are at risk of hypoglycaemia. They should be advised of their risk, given information about the situations that may increase their risk, be aware of the symptoms of hypoglycaemia and know how to take corrective action.

Most patients will be able to recognise the symptoms of hypoglycaemia. These symptoms can be classified as autonomic (caused by activation of the sympathetic or parasympathetic nervous system) or neuroglycopenic (caused by the effects of deprivation of glucose to the brain) (Table 8.1). If able, the patient should confirm their diagnosis by testing their blood glucose, which would be less than 4 mmol/l. (As symptoms of hypoglycaemia may

Table 8.1 Symptoms of hypoglycaemia

Autonomic	Neuroglycopenic
Sweating	Confusion
Palpitations	Visual disturbances
Pounding of the heart	Coordination problems
Tremor	Difficulty with speech
Hunger	Drowsiness
	'Feeling drunk'

be felt if the blood glucose is falling rapidly, the patient should retest after a few minutes even if the reading is above 4 mmol/l. This may happen, for example, if insulin has been injected into a muscle instead of subcutaneous fat.)

The corrective treatment for the symptoms of hypoglycaemia is to immediately eat or drink some fast-acting carbohydrate that can be quickly digested and absorbed, for example five dextrose tablets, 100 ml Lucozade or 150 ml of non-diet carbonated drink (Fig. 8.1). This should be repeated every 10–15 minutes until the symptoms resolve and the blood glucose is above 4 mmol/l (although in reality, the combination of the strong urge to eat and the fear of losing consciousness means many patients overtreat hypoglycaemia).

The patient should then eat some complex carbohydrate (e.g. a sandwich, or their meal if it contains potato, rice or pasta) to maintain the normal blood glucose level. Once recovered, patients should reflect on the possible cause of hypoglycaemia so they can avoid this in the future

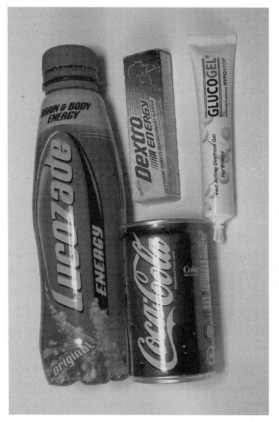

Fig. 8.1 Rapid-acting carbohydrates suitable for treatment of hypoglycaemia.

(e.g. missing meals, or being more active than usual without compensating with extra carbohydrate or reducing their insulin dose).

As the symptoms of hypoglycaemia come on very rapidly, and can then lead to loss of consciousness when not treated quickly, it is essential that all patients at risk of hypoglycaemia (or their carers) carry some form of rapidly-acting carbohydrate with them at all times. District nurses visiting patients at home regularly to give insulin injections should ensure that the patient has some form of glucose available in the house, and within reach if the patient is not very mobile. Often the relatives of the patients have cleared out all sugary foods from the house because the patient has diabetes!

Some patients may not recognise the symptoms of hypoglycaemia or may not be able to take corrective action independently, and so they become drowsy and can lose consciousness. This may happen in the very young child, someone with severe learning difficulties or psychiatric problems, or in people with hypoglycaemia unawareness. This last condition can occur in patients who have had type 1 diabetes for over 20 years, particularly if they have autonomic neuropathy, or in patients who have frequent episodes of hypoglycaemia. These people then have to rely on carers or family members to recognise the signs of hypoglycaemia, and to give treatment. There are two agents that can be helpful in this situation: Glucogel and Glucagen.

Glucogel (formerly Hypostop)

Glucogel contains glucose in a clear gel (Fig. 8.2). It can be useful for patients who are unable to treat their hypoglycaemia independently but it should not be used in anyone who is unconscious or is so drowsy that they have lost their swallowing reflex. The cap of the tube is snapped off and the gel is squeezed into the side of the patient's mouth. The outside of the cheek can be gently massaged to promote absorption through the moist, blood capillary-rich buccal membrane. It should increase the blood glucose sufficiently for the patient to be able to eat or drink some rapid-acting carbohydrate followed by something starchy.

Glucagen

Glucagen is a useful emergency kit for use in the unconscious patient by a trained carer or relative. It is packaged in a distinctive orange box, which contains a syringe ready drawn up with sterile water and a needle in place, and a vial containing 1 mg dried glucagon (Fig. 8.3). The needle is inserted into the vial and the water injected to reconstitute the glucagon within a few seconds. The fluid is then drawn back into the syringe, any air removed, and the contents injected either subcutaneously or intramuscularly. The glucagon takes between 10 and 15 minutes to have an effect (raising blood glucose by increasing glucose output from the liver through glycogenolysis or breaking down of

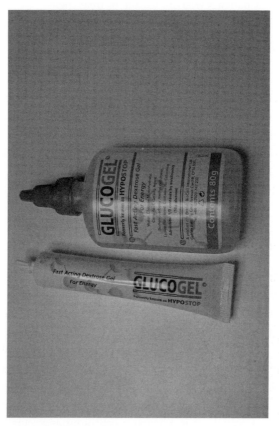

Fig. 8.2 Glucogel.

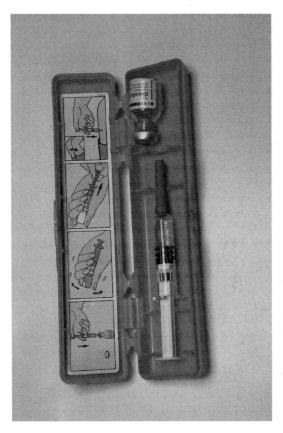

Fig. 8.3 Glucagen kit.

stored glycogen). The patient regains consciousness, usually accompanied by severe nausea and vomiting. Rapid-acting glucose followed by starchy carbohydrate needs to be taken by the patient, difficult though it may be, to prevent a return to the hypoglycaemic state.

It is pointless prescribing this medication to the patient unless his or her regular partner, or a family member, has agreed to use it and has been shown how to draw up and give the injection. It can be helpful for patients who have regular episodes of severe symptomless hypoglycaemia that otherwise would require paramedic intervention.

Painful diabetic neuropathy

It is estimated that about 20 to 40% of people with diabetes will develop diabetic neuropathy, with prevalence increasing with age and duration of diabetes. Its development is related to poor glycaemic control over a prolonged period of time, but the effect of cardiovascular disease is also an important contributory factor. The loss of normal sensation puts the patient at very high risk of developing a foot ulcer, which can have a devastating impact on quality of life, employment, recreation, etc. In about 10% of patients who develop diabetic neuropathy of the feet, the loss of nerve function is accompanied by persistent pain, which may be accompanied by dysthesias (unusual sensations in response to stimulation, e.g. touch). Although the intense pain does improve within about two years, during this period the patient will require a lot of support and the use of various strategies to cope with the pain. As diabetic neuropathic pain is complex in origin, it may not be possible to remove pain completely. Management is focused on reducing pain as much as possible, promoting coping strategies and reducing the risk of physical damage to the numb foot.

Assessment of diabetic neuropathy includes

- when pain occurs (commonly worse at night)
- how sleep is affected
- evidence of depression and mood changes
- pain characteristics (burning, stabbing, shooting, pins and needles, intensity, location, continuous or intermittent)
- sensation using a 10 g monofilament
- vascular status (skin colour, warmth, pulses, hair loss from feet and legs)
- evidence of foot damage (build up of callus, ulcers, deformity, cracked heels)
- history of diabetic foot ulcers or Charcot's arthropathy
- diabetes history
- current glycaemic control (HbA1c and home blood glucose monitoring) and medication
- smoking status
- inspection of footwear and socks/stockings for suitability.

Non-diabetic causes of neuropathy should be excluded:

- malignancy (e.g. bronchogenic carcinoma)
- metabolic (e.g. pernicious anaemia)

- toxic (e.g alcohol or history of working with heavy metals/chemicals)
- infection (e.g. HIV).

First-line treatment

Reducing hyperglycaemia and stabilising blood sugar flux are essential factors in reducing pain. Achieving this may necessitate the patient with type 2 diabetes transferring to insulin, or the patient with type 1 diabetes changing to a more intensive insulin regimen, or even insulin pump therapy.

Non-pharmacological measures include wearing nylon tights in bed, using a bed cradle to keep the blankets off their feet, or putting feet in cold water. Applying OpSite film may reduce pain and contact discomfort.

By definition, these patients will have reduced or abnormal sensation in their feet, so their feet are at high risk of damage from external sources. It is essential that they recognise this and take particular care. This includes daily washing in warm (not hot) water, wearing well-fitting shoes that do not rub or pinch their feet, avoiding warming their feet by sitting close to a fire or putting their feet on hot water bottles etc. They should inspect their feet every day for areas of pressure, redness, blisters, etc., and inspect their shoes for grit and foreign objects before putting them on.

The use of regular simple analgesia such as paracetamol can be effective, especially taken before bedtime.

Capsaicin cream

The active agent in capsaicin cream comes from hot chilli peppers and it can cause a burning or stinging effect. It appears to work by depleting stores of substance P, a local neurotransmitter that is involved in transmitting abnormal pain messages to the brain, in a counter-irritant effect. It has to be rubbed into the skin of the foot four times a day, and its effects often take over a week to be felt, so patients should be informed of this and advised to persevere. It should not be used on broken or irritated skin, or in patients who have skin conditions such as eczema.

Second-line treatment: tricyclic antidepressants

Amitriptyline is one of the most widely prescribed adjuvant analgesics for neuropathic pain (the drug's primary indication is not for pain relief), despite its not being licensed for this use. Tricyclic antidepressants can produce a 50% reduction in pain in about 30% of patients. The precise way in which amitriptyline, and the other tricyclic antidepressants, work is not clearly understood but it is not related to their effect on depression. They may act by blocking activity at muscarinic receptors and alpha-adrenoceptors on nerve cells, which has the effect of reducing sensory nerve function.

Contraindications. Amitriptyline should not be used in patients with severe hepatic impairment, after a recent myocardial infarction or in patients with cardiac arrhythmias, especially those with heart block.

Side-effects. These can be minimised by starting at a dose of 10 or 25 mg, and gradually increasing this to 50 or 100 mg. Taking the drug at bedtime means that the common side-effect of drowsiness is not such a problem, particularly as these patients often have problems sleeping because of the pain. A dry mouth, constipation, hypotension, tachycardia, urinary retention and weight gain are the other common side-effects.

Third-line treatment: gabapentin and pregabalin

Gabapentin was the first oral product specifically licensed for the treatment of neuropathic pain, with significant evidence demonstrating its effectiveness. It should be introduced slowly, starting with 300 mg daily on the first day, 300 mg twice daily on the second day, then three times on the third day, then increase in 300 mg increments daily up to the maximum licensed dose of 1800 mg in a day. The trial data showed patients did need this large dose for the drug to be effective so it is essential that the patient gradually increases the tablets as advised. Patients should also be advised not to use antacids when taking gabapentin as the absorption of the drug is dependent on the amino-acid carrier system, which can be altered by antacids.

Pregabalin is also approved for use in neuropathic pain relief, with trial evidence to demonstrate its effectiveness. It is initiated at 150 mg daily in divided doses, then up to 300 mg daily after three to seven days, then to the maximum dose of 600 mg daily after another week. It should not be used by patients who are breast-feeding, or during pregnancy. Patients who have galactose intolerance, Lapp lactose deficiency or glucose–galactose malabsorption should also not use pregabalin.

Side-effects. Patients may complain of dizziness, drowsiness and ataxia but side-effects are generally less severe than those seen with amitriptyline.

If treatment with either gabapentin or pregabalin needs to be discontinued, it should be done gradually over a week. A lower dose should be used in patients with renal impairment.

Referral for specialist care

Referral to the pain control team. Living with painful diabetic neuropathy is miserable. If the treatments described above do not relieve the patient's pain, then referral to the pain control team should be made for assessment and a variety of pain relief options.

Referral to diabetes foot clinic or podiatrist. Referral should occur for any patient with

- high-risk foot: Charcot's abnormality, ischaemia, absent pulses, neuropathy (NICE foot guidelines)

- active foot ulcer or acute Charcot's foot
- infection of foot or ulcer.

Erectile dysfunction

Erectile dysfunction is extremely common in diabetes, with estimated figures ranging from between 30 and 70% of men. Questioning about sexual function should be included in the annual diabetes review, and the nurse should be conscious of indirect references to this problem that men may make during conversations about their diabetes control.

Vascular damage is the primary cause in about 80% of patients, with or without nerve damage, with 20% being precipitated by psychological factors, particularly depression, which is more than doubled in people with diabetes. It can have a considerable impact on quality of life, with one study demonstrating men with diabetes ranking erectile dysfunction as the third most important complication after blindness and kidney disease.

Assessment of erectile dysfunction will include the following questions.

- Is it a problem with inability to get or maintain an erection or is it a lack in libido?
- Is it important to the patient (and/or his partner), i.e. does he want treatment?
- Is the patient on any medication known to cause erectile dysfunction? Can these be discontinued or substituted?

- Are there any possible endocrine causes (e.g. look for evidence of breast development, reduction in facial hair)?
- How long has this been a problem?
- Did it come on gradually (suggesting an organic cause) or suddenly (more likely to be a psychological cause)?
- Is it a situational problem (i.e. does it occur with one partner but not another)?
- Does he have morning erections (lack of these suggest an organic cause)?
- Is the patient taking nitrates including intermittent glyceryl trinitrate (GTN) spray (this would exclude the use of oral treatments)?

Ideally his partner should be involved in the decision to treat his erectile dysfunction. It can be a shock to his partner if there has not been any sexual activity for years, and he gets effective treatment without warning her (or him).

Factors to consider in erectile dysfunction

Although, ideally, medications that contribute to the problem should be withdrawn, in reality this may be difficult because they include some antihypertensive agents and fibrates, which are important in cardiovascular risk management.

Poor glycaemic control will affect libido if the patient feels tired, and so titration of oral hypoglycaemic agents or insulin, or a change to insulin therapy, will improve this. Balanitis is more common in men with poor glucose control, and the pain from this condition may be a relatively easily treatable cause of erection difficulties. Stopping smoking and reducing excessive alcohol consumption may also be helpful.

The patient should always be asked if he is already using any medication as such medication can be bought through the internet or from advertisements in magazines. He may not know the name of these products but by questioning about the shape and colour, they may be identified as one of the phosphodiesterase type 5 (PDE-5) inhibitors (e.g. blue diamond shape is likely to be Viagra, round brown tablet may be Levitra, and yellow tablet may be Cialis).

First-line treatment: phosphodiesterase type 5 inhibitors

The development of oral agents has revolutionised the treatment for erectile dysfunction, and patients with this condition are now far more likely to discuss the problem, knowing that there is an easy effective treatment available. Interestingly, the first agent, sildenafil (more commonly known as Viagra), was being developed for another indication, and the resolution of existing erectile dysfunction was a side-effect reported by some of the trial patients.

These agents enhance the erectile response to sexual stimulation: this is important to emphasise as they are not sufficient to cause an erection independent of sexual desire.

Treatments for erectile dysfunction at the NHS expense are Schedule 11 drugs and are restricted to men with specific conditions, of which diabetes is one. The prescription should be endorsed with 'SLS' (Selected List Scheme), and patients are permitted one tablet per week.

Contraindications. The PDE-5 inhibitors interact with nitrates and potentiate their hypotensive effect so should not be used in men using these agents, even GTN sprays occasionally. They should also not be prescribed to patients with pre-existing cardiac conditions in which sexual activity is inadvisable, or in men with myocardial infarction within the last 90 days, unstable angina or angina occurring during intercourse. As they are metabolised by the 3A4 isoenzyme of cytochrome P450, they interact with inhibitors of CYP3A4 (e.g. erythromycin, and cimetidine) and so a starting dose of 25 mg is recommended.

Side-effects. Many of the unwanted effects are related to vasodilation in other areas and include headache, flushing, nasal congestion and hypotension.

There are three products: sildenafil, vardenafil and tadalafil.

Sildenafil (Viagra)
An oral dose of 25 mg should be taken an hour before sexual activity (although the effect may be delayed if taken

with food). The distinctive blue diamond-shaped tablet is available in 25, 50 and 100 mg dosage and the dose can be titrated up to the effective dose (which for most men with diabetes is the maximum 100 mg tablet). Sildenafil has a relatively short window of action (several hours). It is effective in about 40% of men with diabetes.

Vardenafil (Levitra)
An oral dose of 10 mg is taken 25–60 minutes before sexual activity; this dose can be increased up to the maximum dose of 20 mg daily. It is effective in about 80% of men with diabetes.

Tadalafil (Cialis)
The 10 mg tablet should be taken at least 30 minutes before sexual activity, and this dose can be increased up to 20 mg if 10 mg does not have sufficient effect (except in men with severe renal impairment). Tadalafil may be effective for up to 36 hours, allowing the potential for erections within this time period (e.g. it can be taken on Friday evening and remain effective until midday on Sunday).

Referral for specialist care

Many diabetes teams run diabetes erectile dysfunction clinics. Specialist advice is required for:

- pyschological cause
- PDE-5 inhibitors are ineffective or contraindicated

- presence of anatomical abnormalities such as
  Peyronie's disease

Other therapies offered by specialists include vacuum
pump, intra-urethral or intra-cavernosal alprostadil and
penile implants.

RELEVANT NICE GUIDELINE

Management of type 2 diabetes: prevention and
management of foot problems. *Clinical guideline* No. 10,
January 2004.

INDEX